Contents

Change, challenge and school nursing

Nicola Madge and Anita Franklin

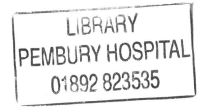
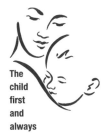

The
child
first
and
always

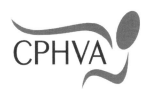

CPHVA

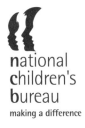

national
children's
bureau

making a difference

The National Children's Bureau promotes the interests and well-being of all children and young people across every aspect of their lives. NCB advocates the participation of children and young people in all matters affecting them. NCB challenges disadvantage in childhood.

NCB achieves its mission by
- ensuring the views of children and young people are listened to and taken into account at all times
- playing an active role in policy development and advocacy
- undertaking high quality research and work from an evidence based perspective
- promoting multidisciplinary, cross-agency partnerships
- identifying, developing and promoting good practice
- disseminating information to professionals, policy makers, parents and children and young people

NCB has adopted and works within the UN Convention on the Rights of the Child.

WA 350

SCHOOL NURSING

Published by the National Children's Bureau, Registered Charity number 258825. 8 Wakley Street, London EC1V 7QE. Tel: 020 7843 6000. Website: www.ncb.org.uk

© National Children's Bureau, 2003
Published 2003

ISBN 1 900990 95 4

British Library Cataloguing in Publication Data
A catalogue record for this book is available from the British Library

Tables

Figures

Acknowledgements

Our first thanks go to all the pupils, school nursing managers and practitioners, and school staff who gave us time and information for this study. As the research is based on what we were told, we could not possibly have managed without their help and cooperation. These respondents have not been named to preserve the anonymity of the study areas, but they may see themselves reflected (accurately, we hope) in the following pages.

Many other people also played an invaluable part in the research. In particular, we received active encouragement and assistance throughout the project from Philip Graham, Pat Jackson, Mary Slevin and Russell Viner who formed our Advisory Group. We are indebted as well to Haydon Bridge High School who helped in the early stages of the study by piloting our pupil questionnaire.

Back at the office, Emma Georgiou, Haddy Njie and Esther Poyer took responsibility for inputting data and transcribing interviews and turned the sea of questionnaires and audiotapes into the quantitative and qualitative information that forms the basis of this report. The friendly help of Emma Moore and Sarah Vaughan, who effected a rapid transformation of our manuscript into this published report at the eleventh hour, was also very much appreciated.

Finally, we would like to thank the Institute of Child Health for their generous funding of the research, and the Community Practitioners' and Health Visitors' Association for their contribution to publication costs.

1. Needs and provision

Health services for young people, according to the NHS Executive (1996), are 'to enable as many children as possible to reach adulthood with their potential uncompromised by illness, environmental hazard or unhealthy lifestyle'. Neither services nor needs, however, remain constant and an examination of both provision and priorities is always timely.

This report is based on research carried out at a time when school nursing services are characterised by both change and challenge. It outlines the findings of a large-scale survey of young people's health needs and perceptions and illustrates aspects of school nursing provision within the same locations. The study does not draw any conclusions for services across the country but uses vignettes to identify the kinds of issues the service is facing. What are the current challenges, what are the obstacles, and what evidence is there that young people's needs are being effectively addressed and met?

Young people and their needs

Most young people these days have good physical health, but some have serious worries or anxieties and many more would like information and support for their health-related concerns. Among other things, they may want to talk to someone or seek advice on personal issues, such as their own relationships, behaviour and health, or on more general issues such as the effects of alcohol and drugs, or contraception and how to get it. They may want to know more about longstanding medical conditions, chronic illness and disabilities, or they may have problems upsetting them or causing their school work to suffer. Certain groups, such as those living in relatively disadvantaged conditions or looked after by the local authority (Kurtz and Thornes 2000), pupils excluded from school and at particular risk of mental health problems, poverty and social isolation (Ofsted 1996), and young refugees and asylum-seekers, may be especially vulnerable.

The following sections provide illustrations from the literature of areas in which pupils' health needs may lie.

General health

Young people who do not suffer from a serious illness or disability may still have specific health problems or just not feel well. The Health Survey for England (Erens, Primastesta and Prior 2001) collected information on the health of a general population sample of several thousand 2 to 15 year olds. A question on illness or injury curtailing normal activities during the previous two weeks was answered by parents for children up to around 12 years and by older children themselves. Overall, 14 per cent of both boys and girls were reported to have had such an illness or injury. Asked to rate their own health, 9 per cent of boys in the sample, and 8 per cent of the girls, said it was fair, bad or very bad. These findings suggested that perhaps one in ten young pupils might have a physical health problem at any one point in time. This was supported by the additional finding that 11 per cent of boys and 9 per cent of girls had seen a GP in the previous two weeks.

A considerable proportion of pupils have chronic medical needs and may face difficulties in mainstream education (Lightfoot, Wright and Sloper 1999; Lightfoot, Mukherjee and Sloper 2001). These comprise a heterogeneous group of children and young people who may have little in common other than that their medical conditions, if not properly managed, could limit their access to education. They include those with illnesses and chronic conditions (e.g. asthma, childhood arthritis, congenital heart disease, cystic fibrosis, diabetes, eczema, haemophilia, ME, sickle cell disease), deteriorating conditions (e.g. childhood cancer, Duchenne muscular dystrophy), injuries and the after-effects of accidents, severe allergies, and disabilities with associated special health needs (e.g. cerebral palsy, spina bifida). The needs of these pupils range from the administration of medication, coping with hidden disabilities, reintegration into school if returning from hospital or home teaching services, keeping up with lessons if repeatedly absent due to ill health, dealing with the uncertainty of a degenerative or deteriorating condition, or the management of severe allergies. The Department for Education and Skills (2001a) recently issued guidance on supporting pupils with severe medical needs and this has been reinforced by Hall and Elliman (2003). Changes are occurring rapidly in this area and new initiatives and programmes are being developed.

Major accidents also contribute to health needs. The 1999 Health Survey for England (Erens, Primastesta and Prior 2001) found that accidents, defined as incidents where a doctor was consulted or a hospital visited, had affected 31 per cent of boys and 22 per cent girls.

Healthy lifestyles

Increasing attention has, in recent years, focused on the promotion of healthy lifestyles among the population as a whole, including young people. Some of the principal areas of concern have been smoking, overuse of alcohol, drug-taking, and poor diets. Many of these appear to affect considerable proportions of young people.

The 1999 Health Survey for England (Erens, Primastesta and Prior 2001) reported that 19 per cent of 8 to 15 year old girls, and 21 per cent of boys of the same age, said that they smoked. This survey also found that 40 per cent of the girls and 32 per cent of the boys reported that they had drunk alcohol. Various recent sources have pointed to the increasing use of drugs by young people. The Department of Health (2002) indicated that 20 per cent of 11 to 15 year olds had used drugs in the past year, and that the most used drug was cannabis. Rates ranged from 6 per cent of 11 year olds to 39 per cent of 15 year olds. Similar findings were reported by Balding (2002). These showed a large increase in the number of boys in their early teens who smoked cannabis: 29 per cent of 14 and 15 year olds last year said they had tried the drug in the previous year compared with only 19 per cent two years earlier.

A national diet and nutrition survey found that one in five 4 to 18 year olds eat no fruit or vegetables at all in a typical week, and many more eat less than one portion of each a day (Department of Health 2000a). Other studies have pointed to the lack of exercise taken by many young people (British Heart Foundation 2000) and how this is particularly pronounced for girls (Haselden, Angle and Hickman 1999). The increasing problem of obesity among children and teenagers (Reilly and Dorosty 1999) has also been highlighted.

Sex and relationships

Sex and relationships education has achieved greater prominence in recent years in response to the falling age of first sexual intercourse, a growth in conception rates and unwanted pregnancies among teenage girls, and a rise in the incidence of sexually transmitted infections.

Coleman and Schofield (2003) compared findings from four studies over the past 40 years (Schofield 1965; Farrell 1978; Johnson *et al.* 1994; Wellings *et al.* 2001) to demonstrate how the proportion of young people who have first sexual intercourse before the age of 16 has increased considerably in even these recent years. Rates remain lower for females than males although they have increased at a more rapid rate.

In relation to pregnancy, the conception rate among 15 to 17 year olds in 2000 was 44 per 1,000 women in this age group, and 8 per 1,000 for 13 to 15 year olds. Just under half of the pregnancies of this older group, and just over half in the younger group, resulted in legal abortion. Sexually transmitted infections among young people are also a cause of concern. There has, for example, been a marked increase in new episodes of genital chlamydia (uncomplicated) among both young males and young females. Such episodes more than doubled among 16 to 19 year-old males and females between 1996 and 2001 in England, Wales and Northern Ireland (Public Health Laboratory Service report quoted by Coleman and Schofield 2003). Sex and relationships education is not only about providing information and skills to avoid unwanted pregnancy and infection, but also about helping to ensure that young people enjoy positive sexual and personal relationships.

Mental health

Mental health, and related behaviours and feelings, present other concerns for pupils at school. At the severe end, there is a small number of young people who commit suicide or make a serious suicidal attempt. Completed suicide rates have remained fairly constant in the past few years and, in 2000, suicide verdicts in England and Wales were returned for two males aged 10 to 14 years and 78 males aged 15 to 19 years. The comparable rates for females were one and 27. These rates are likely to underestimate the scale of the problem as, in reality, many young people receiving open verdicts and verdicts of misadventure may also have taken their own lives (Madge and Harvey 1999).

Non-fatal self-harm among children and teenagers is also an important mental health problem that is rapidly rising in England (Hawton *et al.* 2000) and across Europe (Diekstra, Kienhorst and de Wilde 1995). Estimates based on referrals to hospital following self-harm episodes in England were presented by Hawton *et al.* (2000). These authors suggested that around 19,000 young people between 10 and 19 years are likely to be referred annually to general hospitals in England and Wales following self-poisoning or self-injury. Some 2,000 of these are between 10 and 14 years, and the vast majority are girls. Furthermore, rates seemed to be increasing, especially among girls. These data, nonetheless, refer to hospital referrals and do not include young people who harm themselves but remain 'hidden' within the community. A study, based on self-reported self-harm among mainly 15 and 16 year old pupils at school, found that around 2.5 per cent of young people had carried out some act of self-harm in the past month, 6.9 per cent had had such episodes in the past year, and 10.3 per cent had harmed themselves during their lifetime (Hawton *et al.* 2002). Rates for females were considerably higher than those for males (11.2 per cent of females but 3.2 per cent of males in the past year). This preponderance was confirmed by other recent national data (Meltzer *et al.* 2001) based on parental accounts which indicated that, overall, one in 50 11 to 15 year olds had at some time tried to harm, hurt or kill themselves.

It is difficult to define and ascertain the prevalence of mental health problems more generally, and varied estimates have been reported. A recent review of the evidence (Mental Health Foundation 1999) examined a wide range of information sources and concluded that probably one in five children and teenagers suffers from some kind of mental health problem. It was further estimated that, of these, one in ten has a problem requiring professional help, more than eight in ten have difficulty in getting on with their everyday lives, 12 per cent have anxiety disorders, 10 per cent have disruptive disorders, 5 per cent attention deficit disorders, and 6 per cent developmental disorders. Haselden, Angle and Hickman (1999) reported the findings of a Health Education Authority survey of less severe conditions among over 10,000 young people aged 11 to 16 years in which respondents described symptoms they experienced at least weekly. Irritability or bad temper topped the list for both boys and girls (43 and 42 per cent respectively) followed by difficulties in getting to sleep (33 and 29 per cent), feeling nervous or anxious (34 and 28 per cent), headache (35 and 23 per cent), and feeling low (31 and 23 per cent).

Bullying

Increasing attention has been paid in recent years to the problem of bullying at school and ChildLine received nearly 20,000 calls from children worried about bullying in 2001 alone (Harrison 2002). Elliott (2002) pointed out how most studies suggest that bullying occurs in all types of school. A recent large-scale pupil survey (Balding 2001) included questions on bullying in the last month for Year 6 pupils. Approximately 30 per cent of these primary pupils reported being bullied often or every day: being teased, made fun of, called nasty names, or pushed or hit for no reason, were the incidents most commonly reported. Boys were more likely than girls to report physical bullying, but girls were more worried about going to school because they feared they might be bullied. Many of the incidents reported occurred in the classroom or outside during lunchtime or other breaktimes.

Child abuse and child protection

Information on the prevalence of child abuse is not generally available and estimates vary considerably (Madge 1997). The numbers of young people on child protection registers do, however, give some indication of the size of the problem. In 2001 there were 28,600 young people of all ages on this register in England, of whom roughly equal proportions were aged one to four years, five to nine years, and 10 to 15 years. Smaller proportions of infants under one year of age, and teenagers aged 16 years or above, were also included.

Use of services

There is no clear picture of the number of young people who use the variety of health and related services on offer, and information can be pieced together only from a range of sources. There is also some question about attitudes that young people have towards their own health and the value of health services. Balding (2001) reported that more than nine in ten young people surveyed felt they were in control of their health, and at least a quarter did not think they could influence their health through their own efforts.

So how often do young people turn to services for advice and support and to whom do they turn? It seems that the majority consult their doctor during the course of the year, most commonly for a respiratory problem. Balding (2001) reported that about half of the 42,000 young people surveyed between 12 and

15 years (Year 8 and Year 10 pupils) said they had visited their GP within the past three months, with this figure rising to around 85 per cent for the last year. Few age and gender differences were found although about one in five females, but fewer males, felt quite uneasy or very uneasy during their last visit. Jones *et al.* (1997) reported that about half the young people in their survey had seen a GP in the previous six months and most had seen one in the past year. In general, these young people seemed to attend the surgery about two or three times a year. By around 15 years, about half of all young people were visiting their doctor on their own. Earlier surveys had indicated that both boys and girls were more likely to be at ease with female than male doctors. Churchill *et al.* (2000) found that over one in three consultations with a GP by a sample of 700 pupils in the Midlands were for respiratory conditions. Skin complaints and sports injuries were the next most common reasons for consultations.

This and other evidence suggests that young people are generally happy to visit their doctor, and indeed many wish they could have more time with him or her (Jacobson, Wilkinson and Owen 1994). Nonetheless, young people are not necessarily knowledgeable about how to access primary care services (Kari *et al.* 1997). Jones, Coleman and Dennison (2000) indicated that they would, if possible, choose to see a 'teenage health specialist' at a drop-in facility for all aspects of their health care and, if seeing a GP, would prefer this to be in a clinic especially for young people. On the whole they are most likely to visit doctors for physical complaints and least likely for more 'sensitive' issues. Hawton *et al.* (2002), for example, reported that only 12.6 per cent of 15 and 16 year olds attended hospital following episodes of self-harm and many young self-harmers did not tell anybody about their behaviour. Coleman and Schofield (2001) have, furthermore, raised concern at the small proportion of teenagers who go to their GP with a mental health problem. It is also known that young men attend young people's sexual health clinics far less than young women (Burns 1999; Yamey 1999).

Churchill *et al.* (1997) highlighted the aspects of primary care that seem most important to young people. These authors demonstrated that 'confidentiality' (knowing that if you tell the doctor something, other people will not find out) was most important of all and mentioned by 81 per cent of their sample. Also significant were 'having a doctor who is interested in teenage problems', mentioned by 51 per cent, 'being able to see a doctor on the same day you make the appointment', mentioned by 39 per cent, 'having a special teenage clinic which you can "drop into" if you have a problem', also mentioned by 39 per cent, 'being able to choose to see a male or female doctor', mentioned by

33 per cent, 'seeing the same person each time', mentioned by 20 per cent, and 'being able to discuss problems with a nurse rather than a doctor', mentioned by 17 per cent.

Other services that young people might use for health-related matters include family planning clinics and other providers of contraception. Balding (2001) asked young people about their main source of information about sex, both ideally and in reality. All gender and age groups thought that parents should be the main source of information about sex. Two per cent of the Year 8 pupils and 1 per cent of the Year 10 pupils said that the school nurse was their main source, whereas 3 per cent of males, and 4 per cent of females, in both Years 8 and 10, thought that she should be. Young people were also asked whether there was a local birth control service especially for young people. Knowledge increased with age. As many as three-quarters of the girls in Year 8, but only half those in Year 10, said 'don't know'.

There appears to be little information on young people's perceptions of school nurses and the service they might provide. Balding (2001), however, did ask about the school nurse as one of the people children might possibly turn to. Interestingly, she was mentioned as a source of support only for health problems and not at all for school problems, family problems, problems with friends, career or money problems. Overall, only about one in 20 pupils said they would turn to a school nurse if they had a health problem.

In another study, Oppong-Odiseng and Heycock (1997) asked 253 14 and 15 year olds about adolescent health services including those provided by school nurses. Four in ten – and equal proportions of males and females – said they had used the school nursing service. This was second only to the seven in ten who had seen GPs. Also, 54 per cent said that they knew their school nurse in comparison with 92 per cent who reported that they knew their GP by name or sight. Pupils were most likely to know the school nurse in areas of high or moderate deprivation, and the school nursing service was most commonly used for medical reviews, screening and immunisation. Confidentiality was a key issue for these young people and while 70 per cent thought their GP would treat information confidentially, this was true for 56 per cent in relation to school nurses, 40 per cent for the school doctor, and 59 per cent for other doctors or clinics. Overall, 80 per cent of pupils felt comfortable seeing their GP compared with 64 per cent (three-quarters of the girls but only half the boys) who felt comfortable seeing the school nurse. This finding contrasted with that reported by Eliott, Watson and Tanner (1996) which suggested that pupils seemed to find nurses more approachable than GPs.

Gleeson, Robinson and Neal (2002) reviewed studies looking at teenagers' use of health services and found marked variations in contacts with school nurses. The proportion of young people who reported such contact seemed to range from about 5 to 40 per cent. These authors identified embarrassment, lack of confidentiality, an unsympathetic doctor, inconvenient appointments, an unfriendly receptionist, and poor knowledge of local services, as the main perceived barriers to accessing health services. Factors that seemed to encourage young people to use services were sympathetic staff, the assurance of confidentiality, a doctor of the same sex, a female doctor, a drop-in service, quicker appointments, and taking account of users' views.

The role of school nursing

To what extent does and can the school nursing service respond to the health needs of school-age children, such as those outlined above, and what should be its role and priorities? How have these changed over recent years?

A brief history of the service

Health professionals have been working in schools for almost a century. Concern about high rates of infant and child mortality and infectious diseases, and alarm over 'physical deterioration' among young people, prompted the creation of a universal School Medical Service in 1907. The Education (Administrative Provisions) Act of 1907 gave local education authorities the duty 'to provide for the medical inspection of children immediately before or at the time of or as soon as possible after their admission to a public elementary school, and on other such occasions as the Board of Education direct' (Harris 1995). The focus of the service was on the detection and treatment of poor hygiene and malnutrition and consisted mainly of routine inspections. It immediately came to light that many children had medical issues which impeded their development and education.

The Education Act of 1944 gave local authorities the duty to make arrangements for the medical inspection and treatment of children attending both primary and secondary schools and the Handicapped Pupils and School Health Services Regulations of 1945 led the school medical service to be renamed the School Health Service (SHS). The National Health Service Reorganisation Act of 1973 transferred the statutory responsibility for providing school health services from the Department of Education and Science to the Department of Health and Social Security, and the School Health Service became part of the NHS (National Health Service) on 1 April 1974.

Until 1974 the School Health Service had concentrated on an intensive health assessment and monitoring programme. Since 1974, however, the role of the SHS has increasingly been questioned as the physical health of children has improved and developmental problems are identified by teachers through baseline assessment of school entrants (Cotton *et al.* 2000).

The Court Report (Secretary of State for Social Services 1976) was the first enquiry to examine critically the provision of health care for school children since the inception of the NHS. It recommended specialist training for school nurses to supplement their general nursing qualification, and stressed the need for strengthening the School Health Service with an improved nursing provision so that the school nurse could function effectively as 'the representative of health in the everyday life of the school' (While and Barriball 1993).

Much guidance for health services started to emerge during the 1990s. The Department of Health (1994) recommended that service agreements between school health services and schools should be developed in order to jointly prioritise health targets and jointly plan services. The report stated that such agreements would lead to increased collaboration between health and education staff, and mean a more proactive and effective service that was more responsive to need. The Patients Charter also set out patients' rights and standards of service for the NHS (Department of Health 1996).

At about the same time, the Department of Health and The Queen's Nursing Institute published a document that drew attention to the process of identifying the needs of school-age children, matching resources and needs, prioritising health care and health promotion, and collaboration between health and education services (Bagnall and Dilloway 1996). This brought together evidence on the development of school profiles, the role of the school nurse in health promotion, and the use of skill mix.

Recent developments in school nursing

In some senses the role of school nurses and the service they provide is less proscribed and more ambiguous than at any previous time. Even though school nurses remain the only health professionals exclusively concerned with the full range of health needs of school-age children and their families, and despite much recent detailed documentation on the scope of their remit, what they actually can and do provide is less clear-cut. This is reinforced by the development of a wide range of initiatives to support specific types of health needs faced by young people in which the school nurse may or may not nominally or in fact be involved.

Health authorities retain a statutory requirement to provide health services for children, but there is little legislation specifying what that provision should be. Many expectations of the school nursing service have, nonetheless, been raised. *Saving lives: our healthier nation* (Department of Health 1999b) identified a series of specific targets relevant to young people and highlighted school nurses as key to the public health contribution in this respect. *Making a difference* (Department of Health 1999a) was published in the same year and again provided clarity about what might be expected of this profession. These documents (see panel below) set out a child-centred public health role for school nurses, working with individual children, young people and families, schools and communities, to improve health and tackle inequality. They advised that the role of the school nurse should be developed to enable nurses to lead teams, assess the health needs of individuals and school communities, agree and deliver individual and school health plans, develop multidisciplinary partnerships, and provide a range of health improvement activities.

Saving lives: our healthier nation (Department of Health 1999b) stated that the school nursing service was expected to take the lead on a range of health improvement initiatives including:

- Immunisations and vaccinations.
- Support and advice to teachers and other school staff on a range of child health issues.
- Support to children with medical needs.
- Personal health and social education programmes and citizenship training.
- Identification of social care needs, including the need for protection from abuse.
- Providing advice on relationships and sex education by building on their clinical experience and pastoral role.
- Aiding liaison between, for example, schools, Primary Care Groups, and special services in meeting the health and social care needs of children.
- Contribute to the identification of children's special educational needs.

Making a difference (Department of Health 1999a) outlined how it expected nurses to lead teams, to include nurse and other community and education workers, and to:

■ Assess the health needs of children, and school communities, agree individual and school health plans and deliver these through multidisciplinary partnerships.
■ Play a key role in immunisation and vaccination programmes.
■ Contribute to personal health and social education and to citizenship training.
■ Work with parents to promote positive parenting.
■ Offer support and counselling, promoting positive mental health in young people.
■ Advise and coordinate health care to children with medical needs.

This guidance was followed, in 2000, by a strategy of practice proposed by the Community Practitioners' and Health Visitors' Association, The Queen's Nursing Institute and The Royal College of Nursing (DeBell and Jackson 2000). An agenda for action was outlined to clarify the scope and range of the school nursing service, to explore current issues in the delivery of services, to reach a consensus on a national strategy for the delivery of school nursing services, and to formulate a workplan to address service delivery in line with government policy. The report stated that

> School nursing is committed to the health improvement of children and young people of school age. School nurses recognise that their service has special responsibility for:
> ■ Promoting healthy lifestyles and healthy schools
> ■ Child and adolescent mental health
> ■ Chronic and complex health care needs in children and young people
> ■ Vulnerable children and young people

DeBell and Jackson pointed to a national shift away from universal screening by school nurses to looking at whole population health issues and addressing health promotion and education through interventions that met locally identified needs – with such identification seen as an ongoing process developed in partnership with statutory and voluntary agencies. These authors argued that school health profiling, and the collection of local demographic data and health information at Primary Care Group and Health Authority levels, would help to identify local needs. Health Improvement Programmes

(HImPs) were seen as an important vehicle for this, as was the development of the National Healthy School Standard.

The school nurse practice development resource pack (Department of Health 2001) aimed to provide a framework for developing this school nursing public health role and demonstrated how it involved the following: tackling the causes of ill health; looking at health needs across the school-age population; planning work on the basis of local need, evidence and national health priorities; working within the framework of the local HImP and Education or School Development Plan (EDP); leading or joining multidisciplinary teams and working with other agencies and sectors to plan services and promote well-being; finding out which groups of children and young people have significant health needs; and targeting resources to address these and find meaningful ways to evaluate their work.

Most recently, Hall and Elliman (2003) have reinforced the move towards modernisation of the school health services and the focus on preventive health care, health promotion, and effective community-based response to the needs of families, children and young people. The authors stated

> We believe that the focus should now be shifted away from
> sterile debate about screening, or the functions of school
> nurses and the school health service, towards a radical rethink
> of what children need and how it can best be provided.

They stressed that it should be a service for school-age children, provided at school as well as in other settings, and that the aim should be equity of outcome rather than equity of input. This emphasised that the service should be needs-led and based very much on what young people indicated they would like and need. Partnership working was another priority. These authors recommended extension of drop-in facilities for pupils, highlighted the importance of the school nurse's contribution to the school curriculum and, among other things, pointed to how a more holistic approach could mean she might help to enable young people to 'feel secure and valued, experience increased self-esteem, interact positively with their peers, respond more effectively to pressures over risky behaviour, and make healthy choices'. The National Service Framework for Children is currently under discussion and is likely to take these recommendations further forward.

Working in partnership

The current-day central yet broad role of the school nurse has inevitably meant that she is, in theory at least, relied upon to play a key part in a wide range of specific initiatives and programmes that have been developed in recent years.

The National Healthy Schools Standard (NHSS) is a good example, and the guidance on working towards healthy schools provides a framework for strengthening and delivering the public health role of school nurses within schools. A recent document on the role of school nursing within the NHSS (Health Development Agency 2002) outlined how the service was in an ideal position to provide: confidential one-to-one advice for young people; unique insights into the health needs of the school community; clinical expertise and local knowledge to support school staff; access to information that contributes to a systematic assessment of the health needs of the school-age population through school health plans and other data; and knowledge of and insight into working within wider government policy initiatives. It also recognised that school nurses can make a valuable contribution at a strategic and operational level across all sections of the standard. It acknowledged, nonetheless, that the extent to which school nurses were working alongside the healthy schools programme was highly variable and noted that the barriers to full involvement include competing priorities, a lack of understanding and awareness of the NHSS and/or school nursing on the part of those involved, insufficient training and professional development of school nurses to enable them to carry out their public health role, and the variability in the skills and workloads of school nursing services across the country.

The school nurse can be in an ideal position to promote healthy lifestyles from an early age. *The health of the nation* strategy (Department of Health 1992) identified health targets in five areas (cancers, accidents, HIV/aids and sexual health, mental illness and coronary heart disease) and it has been argued (Bagnall 1997; Osbourne 2000) that, as many of these patterns are established in childhood or adolescence, the best chance of meeting them is through focused health promotion and prevention work with the school-age population via direct access to a named school nurse. The subsequent document entitled *Saving lives: our healthier nation* (Department of Health 1999b) specifically recognised the role of the school nursing service as key to the public health contribution of establishing and responding to the needs of children and young people.

How far is the school nurse these days expected to meet the physical health needs of pupils at school? Kurtz and Thornes (2000) examined the health needs of primary and secondary school children in four different types of location around the country and identified one element of a good service as a designated member of the child health services who had 'sufficient time, the requisite seniority, knowledge, and skills, and designated responsibility to work with each school and its pupils to coordinate and obtain services to meet the health needs of individual children and of the school as an organisation, across all the relevant agencies and services'. While it was recognised that school nurses could, and often did, fulfil this role, it was also noted how at other times they were limited in their ability to do so. The authors concluded that to ensure that they could take on this responsibility, 'significant changes need to be made to their overall numbers, their training, and to the structure of many local child health services'.

A wide range of other strategies has acknowledged the role of school nurses. The service has, for instance, been explicitly linked with raising achievement through the Excellence in Schools programme (Department for Education and Employment 1997), reducing unwanted pregnancies through the Teenage Pregnancy Strategy (Department of Health 2000b), working alongside Personal Advisors in the Connexions initiative (Department for Education and Employment 2000), contributing to the PSHE and Citizenship curriculum in schools, and supporting families (Ministerial Group on the Family 1998) through the improvement of child and family health and well-being. Recent guidance has also stated that 'School nurses have an important role to play in the early assessment and increasingly in assisting schools in delivering effective early interventions for children and young people experiencing mental health problems' (Department for Education and Skills 2001b). The general impression is that the school nurse is, in many respects, expected to be omnipresent and omnipotent.

The service in practice

Expectations of the school nursing service are enormous but what is the reality? Lightfoot and Bines (1996, 1997, 2000) suggested that there were perhaps four key roles of the school nurse: safeguarding the health and welfare of children, providing family support, acting as a confidante for children and young people, and health promotion. They suggested that, in addition, school nurses are increasingly taking on the overarching role of 'health advisor' to pupils, parents and teachers. In practice, however, these aspects of the role are overlapping rather than discrete.

Safeguarding the health and welfare of children

The school nurse safeguards the health and welfare of children in many different ways. Apart from formal duties of health surveillance, such as screening for hearing and vision defects, monitoring growth, immunisation, and carrying out health assessments of new school entrants, she has responsibilities for child protection and vulnerable children. The nurse often works alongside teaching staff in this role, and may act as an advocate for the child, liaise with families and school staff, and play a central role in the network of services for children by referring children to other professionals.

At another level, school nurses may work with schools to develop policies for managing any health needs pupils may have. They might, for example, contribute to a policy on the management of asthma to enable pupils to have access to their inhalers and control their own conditions. Mukherjee, Lightfoot and Sloper (2002) found that provision of appropriate support to pupils with special health needs depended on teachers' understanding of health conditions and their impact on school life, and the contribution of the school nurse in this area can be exceedingly valuable.

Some reports have highlighted how school nurses are able to address the health needs of specific groups. Jackson (1990), for instance, illustrated the role of school nurses in meeting the needs of children from homeless families and identified how this group of children was at risk of weight problems, poor motor skills, dental decay, bedwetting and other behaviour disturbances. Children recently arrived in the UK and their families are another special group and often the school nurse can be their first contact with the health and welfare services.

Recent guidance has increasingly stressed the mental health role of school nurses. Clarke, Coombs and Walton (2003) illustrated what this could mean by outlining a training and consultation model involving psychologists from Child and Adolescent Mental Health Services as well as school nurses. The purpose of the model was to provide a school-based service for adolescents with mental health problems, and it aimed to help the nurses develop their skills in the area so that they could support adolescents to solve their own problems through building up a 'trusting and respectful' partnership. Although the service was used predominantly by female pupils, and although it was not formally evaluated for its impact on young people and their difficulties, the authors considered that it did provide a useful framework for similar projects elsewhere. It also met the recent Mental Health Foundation's (1999) call for young people to have access to services outside a mental health environment.

Family support

The willingness of school nurses to visit families at home, either at the request of teachers or initiated by their own concerns, emerged in the Lightfoot and Bines (1996) study as a potentially important contribution to child health – even if it can be a largely hidden part of their role. Apart from offering emotional support and health advice to parents, school nurses may also liaise with other professionals on their behalf.

Acting as a confidante

Findings of studies have not been entirely consistent, but a number have suggested that pupils often feel they can confide in school nurses. These nurses thus provide an important role for young people unwilling to take their health problems to the GP surgery (Lightfoot and Bines 1996; Bagnall 1997).

School nurses increasingly provide confidential services through drop-in clinics within schools or on nearby premises. One well-publicised example of such a service is the Tic Tac (Teenage Information Centre/Teenage Advice Centre) model which has been replicated in a number of schools. Staffed by a multidisciplinary team that may include GPs, practice and school nurses, health visitors and other health and youth workers, and supervised by a coordinator, the general aim of Tic Tac is to provide a confidential advice and information service for the school population. Tic Tac is also one of the few initiatives of this kind to have been formally evaluated. Examination results have been shown to have improved in schools using Tic Tac and, although difficult to prove this resulted directly from the scheme, the service was widely appreciated by pupils and others (Dawson 2002). Pupils used the drop-in mainly to discuss problems with friends, sex and relationships, and to obtain condoms. Having Tic Tac on site reduced teaching staff time used on pastoral support and allowed more time for the academic side of school.

School nurses have been identified as in a good position to bridge the gap between GPs and other services, and their contribution to teenagers' sexual health has been widely recognised (Day 2000). Sexual health programmes combining education with access to contraceptive services have been shown to be most effective in increasing contraceptive use (NHS Centre for Reviews and Dissemination 1997). An example of a service of this kind, shown to be associated with reduced local teenage pregnancy rates, was illustrated by Wallace (1999).

Health promotion

Lightfoot and Bines reported how school nurses identified classroom-based health education as a key and increasingly important aspect of their work. In this role, they supplied teachers with health related materials, took part in or led lessons, and provided practical experience for pupils such as setting up a mock sexual health clinic (Jackson and Plant 1997). In the view of teachers and pupils, they can make a positive contribution to sexual health education in five main ways (Lightfoot and Bines 1996). First, nurses have expert and up-to-date knowledge that is likely to have credibility in the eyes of pupils. Second, their informal style of health education is considered conducive to discussing sensitive topics. Third, school nurses feel comfortable talking about the human body and are therefore likely to put students at ease. Fourth, nurses were considered to have a non-judgemental approach. And fifth, as outsiders to the school, young people can ask them questions on sensitive or controversial subjects without feeling that there may be repercussions.

There is increasing evidence to suggest that school nurses are undertaking health promotion work within the healthy schools agenda and working within local partnership groups to help meet local health targets, such as within the Teenage Pregnancy Strategy. Most school nurses are trained to issue contraception and others are able to offer first-time contraception and carry out pregnancy tests. Health promotion is also being conducted in new and creative ways. Gunnell (2000) described a six-week health promotion initiative that appeared to be increasingly popular, and was being developed within one of the sites within this research. A babysitting club was set up to enhance young people's parenting and child-care skills through raising their awareness of their rights and responsibilities when babysitting, teaching them about the stages of child development, enabling young people to provide basic adequate child care, providing ideas for play activities, and equipping them with coping strategies and the ability to cope in an emergency or first aid situation.

Health advisor

DeBell and Everett (1998) have argued that many of the services school nurses provide are best described as health advice – and indeed in many areas 'nurses' are now called school health advisors. They are dealing with issues such as children's anxieties about their family and school life, sexual health, eating disorders, drug-taking, depression, exams and personal hygiene, and they are being asked by teachers for advice about children's and young people's emotional and behavioural problems as well as about health education. In this role, school nurses can be well placed to pick up potential problems before they reach crisis point. The many different advisory roles of the school nurse are shown in the following panel.

The different advisory roles of the school nurse

Health advisor to the school as a community
The healthy environment
Health systems and practices
Healthy Schools Awards Schemes
School policies on health
Advisor on communicable disease and infection control

Health-related curriculum and planning
Health need plans for individual children
Negotiated health care plans between school and its health advisor

Health advisor to individual teachers
Health education support for classroom activities
Advisor on the health needs of individual children
Advisor on the management of individual children
Consultant on health concerns about individual children
Advisor on the health of teachers

Health advisor to school-age children and young people
Health sessions for groups and individuals
Health awareness activities
Health information provision
'Listening ear'
Referral to other agencies
Advocate for child to school and/or parent

Health advisor to parents/carers
Health information/advice through informal access to the school nurse
Advice about child health and behaviour-related concerns (Should my child see the doctor?)
Reassurance and guidance about the effects of other children's hygiene and infections
Advice about referral to other professionals
Advocate for parents/carers with the school

(DeBell and Everett 1998)

Lightfoot and Bines (1996) identified the liaison role between different agencies provided by school nurses within the school setting as the most significant function of school nursing.

The present study

The purpose of this study was to look at the health needs of young people and how these are being addressed by changes occurring within school nursing services. A further purpose was to identify the challenges that remain. Research data were collected in two main ways. First, a large-scale survey of pupils at six schools in southern and northern study areas within England was carried out to examine young people's health needs and behaviour as well as their knowledge of the school nurse and her role. Second, semi-structured interviews were conducted with representatives of the school nursing service at different tiers of the service (school nursing managers, team leaders, and nurses with responsibility for particular schools) within the same study areas. These interviews focused on current provision as well as changes taking place within the local service. In one area, ten school nurses also completed diaries of their activities for a randomly selected week. A summary of the research data sources is shown in Figure 1.1. Further details on methodology are provided at later points in this report.

Figure 1.1 Study areas, schools, school nursing professionals and pupils in the study.

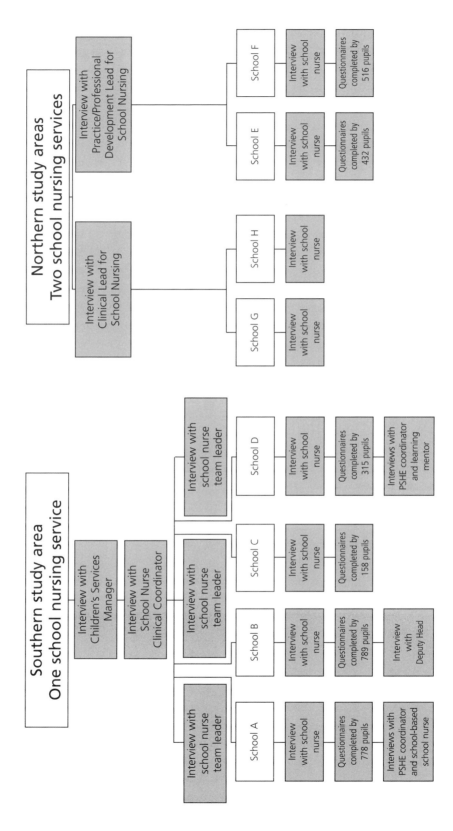

2. The pupil survey

A survey of almost 3,000 pupils at six schools within the two study areas was carried out to find out about young people's views on their own health, their needs for support, and where they would turn for help and advice. Young people were also asked about their contacts with school nurses and their knowledge of the service they provide. Finally, they were asked how they thought their schools might improve pupils' health and how they feel about themselves.

The schools and the pupils

Study schools were randomly selected from all state-maintained, co-educational comprehensive secondary schools within the two study areas. Four schools were chosen in each study area (two in each of the northern study areas) for an initial approach with a further two identified as reserves. All four selected schools in the southern study area agreed to take part in the research as did three in the two northern study areas. One of the reserve schools in the north also agreed to take part. In the event, however, only two of the schools in the northern study area managed to administer the survey in the time available. The final numbers of pupils taking part, together with the location and size of the study schools, are shown in Table 2.1. A total of 2,988 pupils completed questionnaires, and similar proportions of these were male and female.

One of these six schools (School A) had a full-time school nurse employed by the school as well as the health-funded school nurse interviewed. As became apparent, this nurse was not only more visible than the others, but she also appeared to have a somewhat different role in the school. For these reasons, some analyses within this chapter consider School A separately from the rest.

Table 2.1 The schools and pupils in the study

	Study area	Number of pupils in school*	Number of pupil survey respondents			
			Male	Female	Unspecified	Total
School A	South	1156	387	372	19	778
School B	South	1281	388	390	11	789
School C	South	1386	80	78		158
School D	South	1326	148	159	8	315
School E	North	1058	193	226	13	432
School F	North	904	242	264	10	516
Total		7111	1438	1489	61	2988

* not including post-16.

It was not possible to include a representative proportion of young people from black and minority ethnic group backgrounds within the sample, but pupils were asked to say how they would describe themselves. The vast majority (95 per cent) identified themselves as White. Of the rest, 3 per cent described themselves as Mixed, 1 per cent as Asian/Asian British, and 1 per cent as 'any other group'.

Pupils were also asked whom they lived with. Just over three-quarters (76 per cent) stated they lived with two parents and just under a quarter (23 per cent) said they lived with one parent.

Collecting and analysing the research data

An anonymous self-report questionnaire was developed to ask pupils about their health and health needs, their use of existing school and other health services, and their views on both available and potentially available provision.

Once completed, the pupil questionnaires were checked and coded and computer data entry was carried out using the Statistical Package for the Social Sciences (SPSS). Frequencies and cross-tabulations were produced as presented in this report. Statistical analyses to establish significance were conducted as appropriate.

Health and general well-being

Medical problems and general health

Two questions on general health asked, first, whether pupils had a medical problem or a disability (giving dyslexia and asthma as examples) and, second, how they would in general describe their health.

Over a quarter (27 per cent) of the sample indicated that they had a medical problem or disability. The most commonly mentioned conditions were asthma (411 pupils), dyslexia (91 pupils), eczema (48 pupils), hay fever (42 pupils), migraine (16 pupils), diabetes (13 pupils), ADHD (11 pupils), epilepsy (11 pupils) and visual impairment (10 pupils). 'Other' conditions were mentioned by 131 pupils and included both those that were relatively minor, such as an ingrowing toenail, and those that were serious, such as cancer. Age, gender and school did not appear to affect the patterns found. It was not possible from the information given to determine the severity of these reported conditions.

Most pupils, nonetheless, felt that their health was generally good. When asked 'In general, how would you describe your health', 16 per cent said that it was excellent, 41 per cent said it was very good, and 40 per cent said good. Indeed, only 3 per cent seemed to feel that their general health was poor. Males tended to report generally better health: 19 per cent of males, compared with 12 per cent of females, indicated that their health was excellent. Furthermore, and not unexpectedly, pupils who did not have a self-reported medical problem or disability were more likely to report good health than those who did (see Table 2.2).

Table 2.2 Pupils' descriptions of their health according to whether or not they reported a medical problem or disability

	Excellent		Very good		Good		Poor		Bad	
	No.	%	No.	%	No.	%	No.	%	No.	%
Pupils with a medical problem/ disability (N=777)	71	9	309	40	358	46	29	4	10	1
Pupils without a medical problem/ disability (N=2101)	378	18	878	42	795	38	44	2	6	<1

Happiness at school and at home

Pupils were also asked how happy they felt at school and how happy they felt at home. There was a significant correlation between those feeling happy at school and those feeling happy at home, but pupils were still more likely to report feeling happy at home than at school (see Table 2.3). Significant gender differences also emerged, with girls appearing to be happier at school but boys appearing happier at home. Neither happiness at school nor happiness at home was, however, affected by whether or not pupils reported a medical need or disability.

Table 2.3 Pupils who felt happy at school and at home by gender

	Always		Often		Sometimes		Never	
	No.	%	No.	%	No.	%	No.	%
Do you feel happy at school?								
Boys (N=1426)	172	12	650	46	512	36	92	6
Girls (N=1478)	203	14	776	52	439	30	60	4
Do you feel happy at home?								
Boys (N=1432)	723	50	562	39	136	10	11	1
Girls (N=1482)	656	44	599	40	204	14	23	2

Taking care of one's health

Most pupils seemed to think that they took good care of their own health and this was as true of males as of females. Patterns are shown in Table 2.4.

Table 2.4 Pupils who felt they took good care of their health by gender

	Always		Often		Sometimes		Never	
	No.	%	No.	%	No.	%	No.	%
Do you feel that you take good care of your health?								
Boys (N=1429)	411	29	693	48	294	21	31	2
Girls (N=1484)	373	25	770	52	315	21	26	2

Seeking help or information

Pupils were presented with a list of possible concerns or worries. They were asked where they might turn for help or information in these areas and, if relevant, where they had turned in the past.

Where pupils might turn

Ten questions asked pupils where they might seek help or information in relation to relationships with friends, relationships with parents, smoking and alcohol, drugs and solvents, sexual health and contraception, minor illness (e.g. headache), diet and weight, stress, problems at school, and personal appearance. The suggested sources of help and information were telephone helplines, the Internet, a family doctor, a school nurse, a teacher, parents, friends, or somewhere else. Pupils were asked both who they would turn to first and who they might ever turn to.

Parents first, and friends second, stood out as sources of support for pupils and this remained true almost whatever the problem (Table 2.5). Parents seemed especially important in helping with relationships with friends, problems at school and stress, but also for issues surrounding drugs, solvents, smoking and alcohol, as well as appearance, diet and weight, sexual health and contraception. They were also the first people their children would turn to for minor illnesses. Friends were of prime importance for support with relationships with parents, but were also significant for most of the other issues that young people also consulted their parents about. They were not, however, a usual source of support for minor illness, diet and weight, and problems at school.

School nurses were less commonly mentioned as sources of support for any of the problem areas in question. The presence of a full-time nurse at a school, however, made a difference in all areas apart from appearance (Table 2.6). It also made some difference to the reasons why young people might turn to the school nurse. Minor illness was the main reason why pupils at School A used this service, with sexual health, and then drugs, solvents, smoking and alcohol, coming next. Sexual health, followed quite closely by minor illness, was the predominant cause for contacts with the school nurse at the other five schools.

Table 2.5 Where pupils might turn to first, and ever turn to, for help or information

	Telephone helplines	Internet	Family doctor	School nurse	Teacher	Parent	Friend	Other*
	%	%	%	%	%	%	%	%
Relationships with friends (N=2854)								
Turn to first	1	2	1	1	2	48	44	1
Ever turn to	4	5	6	3	17	73	75	6
Relationships with parents (N=2805)								
Turn to first	2	1	2	1	4	30	53	7
Ever turn to	5	3	5	4	13	41	68	10
Smoking and alcohol (N=2759)								
Turn to first	3	2	7	3	2	40	41	2
Ever turn to	7	5	16	7	10	53	58	5
Drugs and solvents (N=2718)								
Turn to first	5	3	11	3	3	39	34	2
Ever turn to	9	5	20	8	10	53	49	5
Sexual health and contraception (N=2712)								
Turn to first	4	3	12	5	1	38	33	4
Ever turn to	9	5	26	14	5	51	48	5
Minor illness (N=2795)								
Turn to first	<1	<1	11	6	3	71	8	<1
Ever turn to	1	1	26	18	12	81	25	3
Diet/weight (N=2721)								
Turn to first	1	2	11	2	<1	62	21	<1
Ever turn to	3	3	22	5	3	71	38	4
Stress (N=2728)								
Turn to first	1	1	5	1	3	49	36	4
Ever turn to	3	2	11	4	9	62	53	6
Problems at school (N=2730)								
Turn to first	<1	<1	<1	1	20	51	24	2
Ever turn to	1	1	1	3	46	75	48	5
Appearance (N=2686)								
Turn to first	1	1	2	<1	1	44	46	4
Ever turn to	2	3	5	2	4	58	61	6

* Most responses within this category consisted of other family members – grandparents, brothers and sisters, or cousins, aunts and uncles.

Table 2.6 Pupils who might turn to the school nurse for help and information – comparisons between School A and all the other schools

	School A (N=778)	All other schools (N=2210)
	%	%
Relationships with friends	5	2
Relationships with parents	6	3
Smoking and alcohol	10	6
Drugs and solvents	10	7
Sexual health	15	13
Minor illness	36	11
Diet and weight	7	4
Stress	6	4
Problems at school	6	3
Appearance	1	2

Nonetheless, even in the two areas of minor illness and sexual health, school nurses were less frequently mentioned as a source of help and information than family doctors – except in the case of minor illness at School A. Apart from parents and friends, the family doctor seemed a popular choice for help and information on health and lifestyle issues. Teachers were seen as an important first source of support for problems at school, and they also had a role in helping with relationship problems and lifestyle concerns.

Helplines, and to a slightly lesser extent the Internet, were also viewed as sources of help or information for these young people, particularly for relationship issues, smoking, alcohol, drugs and solvents, and sexual health and contraception. Other support sources the pupils mentioned were family members such as brothers and sisters, grandparents and cousins, boyfriends and girlfriends, a counsellor, a family planning clinic and a 'weightwatchers' group. Some young people, however, quite specifically said they would not turn to anyone if they had problems or concerns in the various specified areas.

Some interesting differences emerged between males and females, and these were very consistent across problem areas. Boys were significantly more likely than girls to say they would turn to telephone helplines and the Internet, while girls were significantly more likely to seek support from parents, friends and teachers. The only exception was that males were most likely to say they would turn to their parents for help with relationships with parents (presumably they turned to the parent they were not having a problem with). Girls were also more likely to consult school nurses than boys. Interestingly, boys were more likely than girls to seek help from a family doctor.

Recent help or information on health and lifestyle

Pupils were asked next about any help they had sought in the past – either recently or not so recently – and whether the outcome had been very helpful, quite helpful, or not helpful. Overall, and for all problems and concerns combined, pupils were most likely to have consulted parents and least likely to have used telephone helplines (see Figure 2.1).

Figure 2.1 Sources of help and information sought in the past

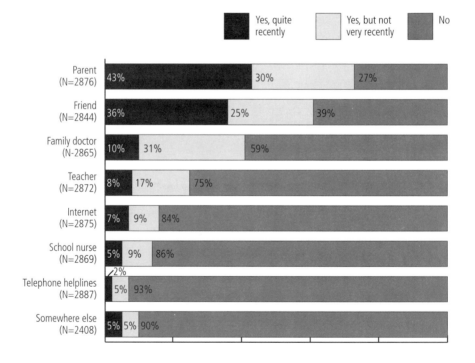

Around one in seven pupils overall said that they had at some time turned to a school nurse. These were much more likely to be girls than boys, and in almost two in three cases the contact had not been very recent. There was also, as might be expected, a difference between schools: more pupils reported contacts with a school nurse at School A than at the other schools (Table 2.7). The most common reasons for seeking help and information were general illness and injury, medication such as painkillers, immunisations, family, friendship and school problems, bereavement, periods and puberty, bullying, eating disorders, weight and diet, sex and sexual health, depression, stress, drugs, smoking and appearance. Pupils at School A were somewhat more likely to mention general illness and medication, but otherwise there were few marked differences between this school and the rest.

Table 2.7 Help and information sought from school nurses in the past – comparisons between School A and all the other schools

	School A (N=747)	All other schools (N=2122)
	%	%
Yes, quite recently	10	3
Yes, but not very recently	23	5
No	67	92

How useful had pupils found the help and information they had received? Parents, friends and family doctors were most likely to have been 'very helpful'. Overall, just over a quarter of the pupils who had contacted a school nurse said she had been 'very helpful' and just over half said she had been 'quite helpful' (Figure 2.2).

Figure 2.2 Sources of support and the level of help received

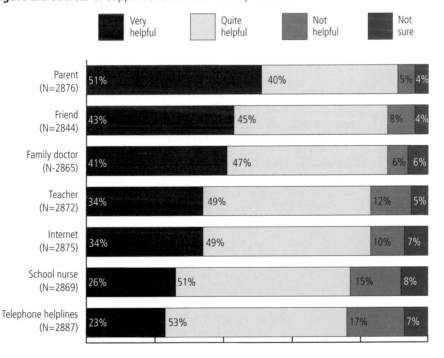

Knowledge of the school nurse

To find out how much they knew about the school nurse(s) at their school, pupils were asked whether they knew who she was and how to contact her, whether they had been provided with any information about her and the service she provided, and whether they had had, or would like, contact with her.

Who she is and how she can be contacted

Not surprisingly, the presence of a full-time nurse at a school considerably increased the likelihood that pupils would know who she was. Thus almost three-quarters of pupils at School A knew the school nurse compared with nearer one in six in the rest of the schools. There was, nonetheless, considerable variation among even these schools with between 10 and 43 per cent of pupils saying they knew her (Table 2.8). Gender differences emerged too. At School A 63 per cent of boys and 85 per cent of girls said they knew who she was, but for the rest of the schools combined the comparative figures were 13 and 20 per cent. Whether or not pupils reported medical problems or disabilities did not appear to affect patterns.

Table 2.8 Pupils who said they knew the school nurse by case study school

	Yes	No	Not sure
	%	%	%
School A (N=765)	74	13	13
School B (N=767)	11	71	18
School C (N=143)	13	64	23
School D (N=299)	43	44	13
School E (N=417)	18	62	20
School F (N=510)	10	77	13

School differences were also found in pupils' knowledge on how to contact the school nurse. At School A, 83 per cent of pupils said that they knew how to contact her, 10 per cent did not know, and 7 per cent were not sure (see Table 2.9). The comparative figures for the rest of the schools were 35, 50 and 15 per cent. Some, but not marked, differences were found between boys and girls. At School A 81 per cent of boys, but 86 per cent of girls, said they knew how to contact the school nurse. At the other schools, 32 per cent of boys and 38 per cent of girls said the same. Once again, having a medical problem or disability did not appear to make a difference.

Table 2.9 Pupils who knew how to contact the school nurse by case study school

	Yes	No	Not sure
	%	%	%
School A (N=761)	83	10	7
School B (N=762)	33	56	11
School C (N=141)	54	33	13
School D (N=294)	43	40	17
School E (N=417)	31	52	17
School F (N=509)	33	49	18

A next question asked pupils how often they thought the school nurse was in the school. Well over half the pupils at School A knew that she was there every day and a further one in three said 'most days'. Many of the remaining 10 per cent of pupils did not know when she was in although some suggested 'only sometimes' or 'never'. Among the pupils in the other schools, well over half overall, and rising to two in three at one school, said they did not know when the school nurse was at school. Those who gave other responses typically said that she came in 'only sometimes'.

Information about the school nurse and her role

To find out more about pupils' knowledge of the school nurse, they were asked if they had ever received information on what she does. Just over half overall said that they had not received any information. Of the rest, similar proportions said the school nurse had spoken in assembly or class, or somebody else had told them about her. One in ten overall said they had seen a leaflet or notice advertising her service (Figure 2.3).

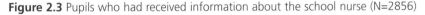

Figure 2.3 Pupils who had received information about the school nurse (N=2856)

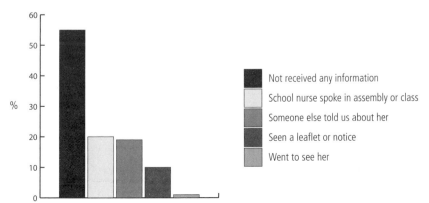

Some notable differences emerged between schools. First, the proportion of pupils saying they had not received any information about the school nurse ranged from 17 to 59 per cent. This did not reflect the presence of an additional full-time nurse at school as the proportions of pupils at School A and the other schools combined saying they had not received information of these kinds were very similar (51 and 53 per cent respectively). Second, there was a division between schools into those where pupils were more likely to have received information from a school nurse speaking in assembly or in class, and those more likely to have been told about her by someone else. Between 4 and 22 per cent of pupils at the schools overall indicated that they had seen a leaflet or notice advertising the service.

An open-ended question asked pupils to say what the school nurse did at school and invited them to write down as much as they knew. Many different answers were given. By far the most common, and mentioned by just over half the pupils, was 'helps with problems', 'gives advice', 'counselling' or a similar answer. Help with illness and injuries came a reasonably close second. All other possibilities were mentioned much less often but talking in lessons, injections and vaccinations, gives out medication, contacts parents and sends you home if ill, first aid, nothing, and helps with sexual health, contraception and pregnancy testing, were the most common of these.

Pupils in contact with the school nurse

Pupils had already been asked if they had sought help or information from the school nurse (see Figure 2.1) and they were now asked if they had had *any* kind of contact with her. Those who had not were also asked if they would like some contact. Not surprisingly, far more pupils had had any type of contact with her than had specifically sought support. Overall, one in three said yes to this more general question and the rest said no (Figure 2.4).

Figure 2.4 Pupils who had had contact with the school nurse (N=2773)

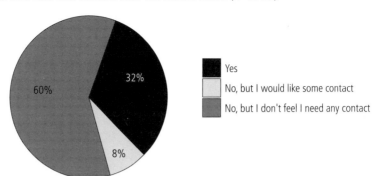

These figures, nonetheless, concealed wide variation between schools and in particular the striking, and expected, differences between the school with a full-time school-based nurse and the rest (Table 2.10). While three-quarters of pupils at the first of these schools had had contact with a nurse, the proportions in the other schools ranged between 5 and 29 per cent.

Table 2.10 Pupils who had had contact with school nurse – comparisons between School A and all the other schools

	School A (N=725)	All other schools (N=2048)
	%	%
Yes	75	17
No, but I would like some contact	2	10
No, but I don't feel I need any contact	23	73

Vaccinations and injections, class lessons, and health concerns were the main reasons for seeing the school nurse (Figure 2.5). Other things listed by pupils under 'something else' included counselling, bullying, general problems, pregnancy testing, stress and 'personal'.

Figure 2.5 Pupils and the reasons for their contacts with the school nurse (N=777)

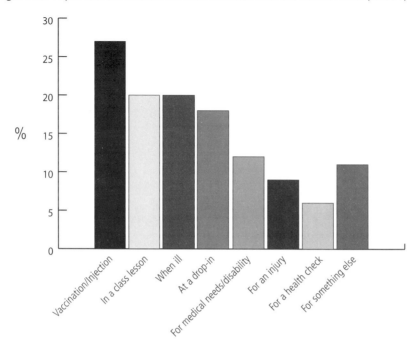

Although most of the pupils who had not had contact with the school nurse said they did not feel that they needed any, 8 per cent overall said they had not had any contact but would like some (Figure 2.4). The proportion of pupils requiring some extra support of this kind was higher in the schools without the additional full-time nurse. Rates varied between 2 and 13 per cent of pupils in individual schools. There were almost equal proportions of boys and girls among the 222 pupils who indicated they would like contact with a school nurse, and nearly 3 in 10 of these pupils had stated that they had a medical need or disability.

There seemed to be a high level of general satisfaction about the contacts that pupils had had with school nurses. Of the 889 pupils who reported a contact, 681 (77 per cent) said she had been helpful and 108 (12 per cent) said she was unhelpful. The remaining 100 (11 per cent) did not say what they thought. Few differences were found between School A and the rest in this respect.

Current needs for help or information

Health and lifestyle

Current needs for help or information on health or lifestyle were explored next. Pupils were asked whether or not they had any such needs and a small proportion of pupils, about one in 12, indicated that they did. Almost two-thirds of these were female, and nearly two in five reported a medical need or disability.

A range of needs was identified by this small group of pupils. Healthy eating or weight problems were most often mentioned, followed by specific health issues such as asthma and dyslexia, family problems, general issues such as relationship problems, and bullying. Other areas included puberty, appearance, getting fit, suicide, self-harm, help with an injury, eating disorders, drugs, smoking, sexual health, exam stress, and death or illness in the family.

The best places to get help or information

Pupils were asked where they would most like to get help or information from somebody, such as a school nurse, trained to deal with young people's health and worries. Almost half gave one preferred source, one in five mentioned two sources, and the rest mentioned three or more.

The most popular response, given by almost half the pupils, was home. This no doubt reflected many young people's preference for help and information from parents. The doctor's surgery, followed by school, were the next most common answers (Figure 2.6). Considerable numbers of pupils also had preferences for the other suggested places for support such as hospitals, drop-in centres, telephone helplines, youth clubs, and Internet cafés.

Figure 2.6 Where pupils would most like to get help or information (N=2652)

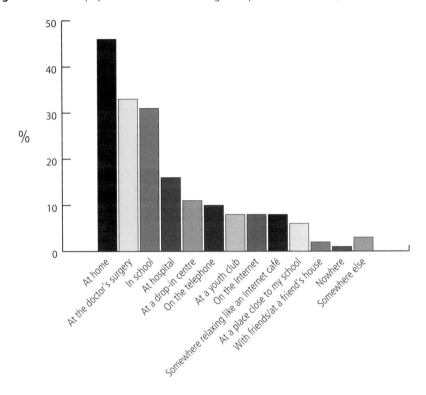

Pupils' responses were examined by gender and some interesting findings emerged. There were no marked differences between boys and girls in their preferences for help and information at home, the doctor's surgery, hospital or a youth club, but there were significant differences for school, drop-in centre, telephone and the Internet. Consistent with the earlier findings, girls were more likely than boys to say they would prefer to receive support from the first three of these sources while boys were more likely to prefer the fourth.

More about schools

Someone to turn to at school

To set the findings on school nurses in perspective, pupils were also asked if they felt there was a member of staff they could turn to at school if they had a worry or concern. Within the sample as a whole, almost half the pupils (49 per cent) mentioned someone that they could turn to, one in three (32 per cent) said there was nobody, and one in five (19 per cent) were not sure. The main members of school staff mentioned were form tutors or heads of year. Girls were significantly more likely than boys (57 compared to 43 per cent) to feel there was someone at school to turn to.

How schools could improve the health of pupils

At the end of the questionnaire pupils were asked to write down three things they thought their school could do to improve the health of its pupils and how they feel about themselves. Almost 2,000 pupils answered this question. Over half of these made two suggestions for improvements and over 600 listed three.

A wide range of suggestions was made, and the top ten responses are shown in Table 2.11. Healthier food, and cheaper food and drink, were the most frequent response, but someone to talk to or provide information and support came second. Better toilets, more sporting equipment and opportunities, and more information on health education issues came next. It is interesting to note that the school nurse could potentially have an impact in about half of these 'top ten' areas.

Table 2.11 The 'top ten' things the school could do to improve the health of its pupils and how they feel about themselves

	Number of pupils (N=1953)
	%
Healthier food/cheaper food and drink	547
More nurses/nurse in more regularly/someone to talk to (e.g. drop-in/counsellors)	410
Cleaner/improved toilets	371
More PE/more sports facilities, equipment and opportunities to play sport and exercise/go swimming	235
More information on health, life, sex education	215
Cleaner school/canteen	215
More understanding by staff of being ill/needing help/look out for pupils more	176
Reduce bullying	156
More information on what the school nurse does	117
Stop the smoking in school	117

To summarise

The pupils who took part in the survey generally said they were healthy and felt they took good care of their health. Nonetheless, over a quarter suggested they had a medical problem or disability of some kind. Overall they were most likely to consult parents or friends if they had problems or concerns, but might turn to family doctors or teachers for certain kinds of worries. The school nurse was not usually who they would turn to first, but pupils might see her as a source of help and information – particularly for minor illness or sexual health matters. There were marked gender differences in help-seeking behaviour with girls preferring to sort out their difficulties through personal contacts and boys seeking more anonymous means.

Except in the study school with an additional full-time nurse, only a minority of pupils knew who the school nurse was. Most did not know how to contact her or how often she was in school, and the majority said they had not received any information on who she was and what she did. About one in three overall reported some contact with the school nurse (this varied between schools, particularly those with and without a full-time nurse), and most of those who did had found her helpful. A small proportion of pupils indicated that they had not seen a school nurse but would like to. Other pupils said they had current needs for help and information. Issues around healthy eating and weight were most often mentioned. Home was the preferred source of help and information for these young people, and the doctor's surgery and school came next.

Young people made many different suggestions about what schools could do to improve pupils' health and how they felt about themselves. Providing healthier and cheaper food and drink came top and reinforced how diet and nutrition are matters of considerable concern to secondary school pupils. More school nurses and other people to talk to was something else the young people said they would like.

3. School nursing in transition

School nursing services across the country are highly variable and, almost everywhere, in a period of rapid change. This chapter presents snapshots of services in three locations – one in the south of England and two smaller neighbouring areas in the north – to provide examples of the philosophy behind current change and challenge and the meaning of this change in practice. The accounts are based on interviews with people at different levels within the school nursing service who have differing levels of expertise and spoke for themselves as much as for the service more generally.

What follows is not, therefore, an authoritative account of current school nursing practice but rather brief vignettes of provision in the study areas from which the young people participating in the pupil survey were drawn. Any points of comparison between what young people and school nurses* said are highlighted in Part 4.

The southern study area

This area as a whole was geographically diverse with urban, rural and seaside areas. It was divided into five large school nursing team patches characterised, according to its Action Plan 2002–2005, by widespread pockets of deprivation, large numbers of refugees and asylum-seekers, looked after children and young people on child protection registers, and high rates of teenage pregnancy. The population included around 109,000 pupils in state primary, secondary and special schools, and there was a shortage of schools in some localities.

Interviews were held in this area with the Children's Services Manager, the School Nurse Clinical Coordinator, three of the six school nurse team leaders, and the school nurses attached to four randomly-selected case study schools.

* The term school nurse is used interchangeably with other job titles.

These interviews explored the issues confronting the service at the present time, current priorities and change, and the services provided within the case study schools. Diary entries illustrated the tasks undertaken by ten nurses in one locality during one week. The following sections are based on information from these sources.

The philosophy of the service

A public health role characterised the philosophy and operation of the school nursing services in this area and dictated the changes that were occurring. The contrast between this approach and the more traditional health delivery model was explained by the Children's Service Manager.

> 'Within the health delivery model, child protection means knowing a child is at risk, attending case conferences, being an advocate for the child, helping to decide the child's future and then helping to support the child and the family. In the public health model, it's around prevention of that happening in the first place. Even as far back as setting up a breakfast club at school. It is around prevention and picking up issues early. And not just prevention with the individual but prevention of groups of young people. So it's targeting a school where there is a high number of children at risk.'

A school nurse team leader outlined how this was put into practice and heralded a new way of working. She gave the example of a babysitting course at a secondary school set up to help pupils develop parenting skills and, hopefully, reduce their risk of teenage pregnancy.

> 'We're preventing people from falling in the river instead of trying to pull them out the other side.'

The role placed a great emphasis on partnership with agencies and other significant people. It meant training and supporting teachers and helpers in schools so they could, in turn, support young people. It was also about helping parents and carers to help their children. The service had moved from a reactive response to proactive health promotion and parent empowerment as illustrated by the shift from checking for headlice to encouraging parents to monitor their own children.

Nurses enlarged on the multi-agency work they were involved in. As well as liaising with a range of different professionals (e.g. teachers, paediatricians, psychologists, child psychiatrists, SENCOs, EWOs, health visitors, speech therapists, occupational therapists), they mentioned involvement with initiatives (such as the National Healthy School Standard, Children's Fund projects, Quality Protects, Sure Start, Homestart, and HImPs), their role in helping to meet official targets (e.g. targets for inclusion, attainment, and teenage pregnancy), and the way they were taking on board guidelines on a public health strategy. Participating in local schemes, and linking in with community services (e.g. child and adolescent mental health services, social services, hospitals, GP practices, voluntary agencies) were also cited.

Partnership working brought its own problems. The enormous number of current initiatives impinging on pupil health could mean blurred boundaries and considerable overlap between what different people and groups were attempting to do. This was an inefficient use of resources and could be overwhelming for all concerned – especially schools.

Despite a general move in the direction of a public health model, there remained some differences of ideology and perspective within the area as a whole. The impact of bringing together two nursing services, with very different practices and ways of working, was still apparent. One of these areas had, in a sense, been more traditional and viewed universal screening and child protection as among its key tasks, while the other had placed a lesser emphasis on these aspects of the role but greater stress on health education and preventative work within schools. One team leader said:

> 'People did work very differently and still do work very
> differently. As an outsider coming in, I would say very clearly
> there's quite a lot of rivalry and rankling. You know, "this is
> how we do it here and this isn't how we do it here".'

Some nurses felt there was still a strong case to be made for meeting basic health needs such as screening for vision, hearing, height and weight, as well as enuresis and headlice infestations.

> 'It's no good going out and doing all these high powered
> things if you've got a whole raft of children underneath
> whose general basic health needs aren't being fulfilled. In
> [one area] that's what we feel as a team needs to be
> happening. It's great to have all sorts of behaviour

> modification and going out to do specialist clinics but if
> you're not looking at the general basic health needs of
> children then I think we've lost the plot.'

Overall, and despite some differences between areas and teams, the generally accepted philosophy throughout the area appeared to be that it was best to carry out a comprehensive pupil assessment at initial school entry and then target services as issues became apparent. A team leader thought the service had rapidly become more proactive, less universal and more target-led.

> 'I would say up until a couple of years ago school nurses
> were still entrenched in a very sort of generic all-singing,
> all-dancing role. You know, I could do a bit of everything.
> The shift, and I'm really pleased with the way things have
> shifted, is that we now look at the team and individuals to
> see what attributes and skills they've got that they can bring
> to the team.'

The school nurses and their caseloads

At the time of the study interviews (around June 2002) there were a total of 11.86 full-time equivalent school nursing posts at F, G or H grades, 9.26 posts at D and E grades, and 2.76 posts at A, B or C grades for a school population of about 109,000 pupils. Full-time equivalent in these cases implies employment on a 45 week term-time basis. These nurse to pupil ratios were below those recommended by the Court Report (Secretary of State for Social Services 1976).

Almost all nurses expressed a general frustration with the size of the caseloads. One of the team leaders with 56 primary schools, six secondary schools and two special schools in her patch said:

> 'I'm not feeling too happy today about the number of
> school nurses. You know, we're feeling very stretched and
> I know everybody says that but there are just some days when
> I think this is ridiculous, this is bizarre, there's so much work
> to do. And I'm having one of those days.'

Another team leader described the workload of her team:

> 'We have three trained nurses who each have about 18 to 20
> schools. One has the vulnerable children specialism and has
> five secondary schools, and the others have two secondary
> schools as well as the primary and special schools. They act
> as named school nurses and deal with child protection, look
> at service agreements, SENCO liaisons, programmes of care
> for children with special needs, and liaise with the
> management team to look at things that specifically go on in
> that school. The staff nurses would be doing the day-to-day
> work with the children on a routine basis and following up
> the issues with parents. They would have certain schools
> allocated to them. One staff nurse has a specialism in family
> planning, another one to come will be doing enuretic
> clinics, and another does the domestic violence forum.'

It was not only large caseloads but also practical difficulties that the school
nurses had to cope with. A third team leader said:

> 'It's a high number, a very big geographical area and there's
> a slice of our patch which is actually part of another PCT. It's
> very muddled.'

Changes were, however, occurring and there was a move away from school
nurses having their own special caseloads. Skill-mixing within nursing teams was
being introduced so that each school had a named nurse but also used the
services of other members of the team as appropriate. Teams comprised nurses
with different skills and expertise to meet a wider range of needs. There might,
for example, be one nurse with special responsibility for special health needs,
another for adolescent health (including sexual health), and another for
vulnerable young people (e.g. child protection and child deprivation). New
specialisms for the future were likely to include pupils in transition, emotional
health, and immunisations. Some members of teams, and particularly nurses at
the lower grades, would however remain generic.

Skill-mixing is most effective where there are adequate resources and a good
range of skills within teams. In practice, and as illustrated at the case study
schools, school nurses rarely had time to visit schools not on their caseloads.
And, within their own schools, they tended to focus on their areas of interest
and specialism. In reality this meant that certain health concerns received

greater attention than others. According to one school nurse, family health and sexual health services were provided more comprehensively than others, except for immunisation, because most school nurses had been trained in these areas.

The nurses at school

Differences in provision and profile were evident among even the school nurses attached to the four study schools. Three of these nurses had an F grade and one a G grade post. Three of the four had degrees and all had undertaken a range of training courses. They had worked at the present schools for between five months and five years and had responsibility for differing numbers of schools as well as different caseload arrangements, i.e. one had a 'corporate caseload' shared with other nurses.

There was marked variation in the number of times the school nurse would typically visit the school. One said she visited nearly every day, another said she had been about three times in the previous month (and acknowledged that she was not a high level resource for this school), a third – working at a school where there was another full-time nurse – said she had visited about eight times in the past month (once a week for the drop-in, once a week for a health education session, and occasionally for other matters), and the fourth said she had visited more than ten times in the current month (once a fortnight for the drop-in, and at other times to see pupils or parents).

Asked how many of the pupils would know who she was, two school nurses said about half, and one said she hoped it would be half but suspected it was rather fewer. The fourth said probably only about one in five pupils would know who she was.

Priorities in theory

The public health model prescribes a way of working rather than the content of the tasks undertaken. How did the nursing service in this study area aim to provide a needs-led service?

The Children's Services Manager outlined what happened in theory. She explained how the service worked in partnerships to understand the key targets in the area. Clear Partnership Strategic Agreements for reducing teenage pregnancy, for example, existed in two of the six areas, and school nurses had to take these on board. Other agreed targets were about raising attainment where the school nursing role related to health and emotional health, and encouraging children to stay at and attend school.

Other factors, too, influenced how priorities were set and how the school nursing service actually operated. First, and very much in line with the public health role, resources were targeted in areas of greatest need. This meant looking at local profiles as well as other local knowledge and information. The general strategy was to support schools with higher levels of deprivation. As one team leader put it:

> 'We say we've got 20 per cent of schools where we need to give 80 per cent of our time, and 80 per cent of schools where we need to give 20 per cent of our time.'

This did not necessarily mean targeting all the most needy schools. A failing school might, for example, already have high levels of support from other services and initiatives. School nurses would not have a significant role in these and their limited resources might be better used where there was a lesser degree of need but a greater lack of support.

Another consideration affecting priorities was the need to meet statutory obligations in the areas of immunisation and child protection. Although nurses unanimously recognised these priorities, they also pointed to how they could interfere with other aspects of their role.

> 'It's certainly our role to lead and certainly school nurses are experts in the leading of the campaign but they shouldn't be the sole provider. So it just knocks you back. It took us three years to get over the MMR campaign and catch up on things like school entry screening and other immunisations.'

The concentration of resources on immunisation often meant that proactive work, such as drop-in sessions, after school sessions, and working with parents, had to stop or was seriously curtailed. This could damage relationships with schools, sometimes in the longer term. To respond to these difficulties, the area's Action Plan for 2003–2004 mentioned the aim 'To research and develop immunisation teams, so that the school nursing service is not totally disrupted by mass immunisation programmes'. Meeting statutory requirements to attend child protection conferences or write reports could also be time-consuming and reduce the time available for other initiatives.

Service level agreements were highly important in determining the school nursing role in individual schools. Many things, such as providing emergency contraception and pregnancy testing, could be provided only with such agreements. The service had produced guidelines for schools on developing sexual health service level agreements with the school nursing service which outlined the skills of school nurses, and the conditions under which they could work best in schools. These offered a number of possible sexual health 'menus' – although schools and nurses could design their own if they preferred – ranging from high to low school nurse involvement. In practice it seemed that many schools were working in this direction. Of the four case study schools, one had a service level agreement in place, two were awaiting final agreement, and one was at an earlier stage of discussion.

Priorities in practice

Not surprisingly, nurses indicated that determining priorities was easier in theory than in practice. Despite guidelines and an ideological perspective, it was easy to become sidetracked.

> 'We should probably have a much more consistent, coherent
> priority setting really. I'm not happy about the way that it is
> but I hope it's something that we're working towards.'

The interests and specialisms within the school nursing teams had a strong influence on services provided. There was clear evidence that individuals could drive particular areas forward in their areas of interest and expertise. Some nurses also pointed to the significance of inheriting commitments from nurses previously in post.

Schools themselves also made a difference – in both positive and negative ways. Some were very enthusiastic about school nursing services while others, for various reasons, were less so. This was illustrated by the case studies. The nurses working at two of these schools said they were made very welcome and had a high level of cooperation with staff. The assistant head at one of these was present at the interview and said the school had really wanted the school nurse and was keen for her to be seen as part of the staff. In the third of these schools, which also had its own full-time school-based nurse, there was clearly a good and mutually supportive working relationship between the two nurses, and pupils had the choice of two different people to approach for health-related concerns. In the fourth of these schools, however, the nurse reported that the school had a good pastoral support system and so did not actively seek the school nursing service and involve it in planning as much as some other schools.

Nurses were, however, aware that they should not over-respond to schools that demonstrated enthusiasm for their support. As one put it:

> 'A lot of the privileged schools know very well how to shout. So we are conscious that we don't just respond to the people who shout loudest.'

Sometimes, indeed, it was very much a question of convincing schools that school nurses had something to offer.

> 'I think that if the need is there then we just have to make inroads. A secondary school that we have had to work quite hard in wants to come and talk about the morning after pill next week. So it works. You just have to keep being there, keep offering, keep reminding them. Yes, a dripping tap.'

With limited resources, nonetheless, setting priorities was never the whole story.

> 'With the funding that we've got, and the hours that we've got, at the moment we can really only scrape the surface.'

Meeting needs in the case study schools

The case studies provided more detail on the ways that nurses worked with individual schools. They revealed very different patterns that depended on the nurse herself, the school, the local priorities, and available time and resources.

Immunisation was, for all, a priority, although one nurse had not been in post long enough to know how it worked in practice. Two indicated that this role had taken up an enormous amount of time, and one indicated that it had been the best means of making contact with the school. Another said that the process of immunisation was organised very efficiently in her school and had not been a highly onerous task. One nurse suggested that immunisation would be better carried out by lower grade nurses. Child protection, too, was an important aspect of provision for all nurses. Making referrals and attending case conferences were a significant part of this role.

No systematic screening was carried out by school nurses in the area, and there was also little emphasis on medical issues such as minor accidents and injuries. Mental health was highlighted as an area presenting a real need. This was dealt with, in the main, through the drop-in sessions (see below).

An important aspect of the public health role for school nurses is their contribution to the school curriculum. The four case study schools received rather different input in this respect. Two of the four nurses did not contribute to any lessons – one said she had never been asked to and the other indicated that she hoped to in the future once the service level agreement had been drawn up. Of the two who did, one was responsible for covering health and sexual health within Sex and Relationships Education, and the second contributed on a regular basis. She carried out a rolling programme covering puberty with Year 7, relationships with Year 8, contraception with Year 9, sexually transmitted infections with Year 10, and general male and female health issues, and how to access services, with Year 11. Nonetheless this involved only one session with each year group and the nurse said:

> 'To me, that isn't very much when you are talking about health.'

Providing a 'listening ear' to pupils was another important role. School nurses held drop-in sessions at three of the four case study schools, and the fourth had in the past. One of the existing drop-ins operated once a week and the other two operated fortnightly, although one nurse would have liked to be able to run hers weekly. Besides at drop-in sessions, nurses saw pupils on a one-to-one basis as required. According to one nurse, seeing pupils informally and flexibly was more effective and a most important and most time-consuming aspect of her work. She felt she was meeting a crucial need as young people had nowhere else to go locally, other than their GP, for contraception, emergency contraception and pregnancy tests.

A recent development in the study area had been to set up a mobile phone service. Each nursing team had two telephones and pupils could send text messages between 9 a.m. and 5 p.m. to seek advice or information. This initiative had proved highly successful. It had reduced the numbers of pupils attending drop-in sessions and had helped with workloads. The scheme would almost certainly be extended within the locality.

Although school nurses were able to offer pupils only 'tier one' support, and did not provide more formal counselling, they stressed the value of what they were able to do:

'I feel that they haven't got anywhere else so it is a very
important part of my work. I am not a counsellor by any sense
of the word. However we have done brief solution focus therapy
training and that's what we use. That works quite effectively.'

Nonetheless, they were not reaching all pupils and boys, in particular, were
being missed. One nurse emphasised how she almost always saw girls and had in
fact only ever seen two or three boys. Girls were much more willing to talk over
their problems with a school nurse and there was a general awareness of the
need to find ways to provide similar support for boys.

Monitoring and record keeping

Various records were kept systematically across the study area as a whole. First,
details of all screening and immunisation were kept on a central child health
computer. Second, child health records were kept centrally for all pupils, and
included notes on their contacts with the school nursing service. Third,
information from these child health records was extracted and included on the
ComCare database. This monitored the reasons for contacts with pupils, and
where contacts had occurred, and provided some evidence of the school nursing
service in practice.

Pupil health records did seem to be regularly maintained and were drawn on in
relation to child protection or mental health issues. Nurses also said they were useful
for other nurses taking over responsibility for a child. They did, however, have their
limitations. While providing a helpful picture of local provision and services
provided at schools, they failed to take account of many activities that did not fit
within their remit. They could also provide misleading comparisons. For example:

'A lot of things that we spend time doing aren't actually
accountable. If you do a school assembly it looks like you do far
more contacts than someone who has more administrative
duties and fewer contacts with individual children. As a team
leader there are some weeks when I don't see any children. I
think that's very disappointing really. I only go to meetings
about them.'

In addition to keeping their own records, nurses may play a part in the
development of school profiles describing the school population and identifying
numbers of pupils with particular health needs, on the child protection register,
in receipt of free school meals, and so on. They may also contribute to local and
community profiles.

The impression given by school nurse team leaders was that school health plans and school profiles were not consistently kept and updated. One suggested these had probably been up to date in her patch until about a couple of years earlier but that no fresh profiling had been done since then. The matter had been under discussion, but time constraints had meant that nothing further had been done. A second team leader indicated that she had not undertaken a formal school profile until very recently when a variety of data sources (on free school meals, the proportion of pupils with special needs, etc.) had been used to identify the most needy schools. A third team leader reported that her team was looking at the Huddersfield model (see page 75) and had begun to profile schools and their pupils. This process had, however, been interrupted by the immunisation programme.

Audits were regularly carried out in the study area to provide a basis for service planning. The School Nurse Clinical Coordinator said that the policy was to 'audit, evaluate, and re-audit' to ensure that policy and practice were evidence-based. These audits were carried out on many different subjects, for example, child protection policies, or record keeping, and the results passed to Clinical Governance for ratification. Their outcomes were used to update standards and practice guidelines.

A number of general issues were raised by nurses on monitoring and record keeping. First and foremost, there was a concern that any information collected should be meaningful and useful in directing or evaluating service provision. Such data needed either to be able to demonstrate outcomes, such as in relation to government targets, or to be framed so that it could dictate service needs and their focus. In practice records were very time-consuming to maintain, and those such as school profiles had not demonstrated much added value over and above the local knowledge and understanding nurses already had. Furthermore, as one team leader pointed out, the pupils in most need of support do not necessarily attend the most 'deprived' schools.

School nurse diaries

Ten school nurses in the southern study area completed diaries of their activities over a week-long period to provide a more detailed look at what their work entailed. Their entries for Monday (the first day that was recorded for the present research purposes) during this week are presented in Figure 3.1. These may or may not have been typical of their normal working patterns. It is important to note, too, that these nurses did not all have similar roles and one (Nurse C) was of a considerably lower grade than the others.

Figure 3.1 School nurse diary entries for Monday

TIME	LOCATION	ACTIVITY	CONTACT WITH	COMMENTS
NURSE A				
9.00	School.	Well Persons Talk on Breast and Testicular Examination.	Sixth form head and 30 sixth form pupils.	Lesson observed by school nurse working with vulnerable children.
10.00 to 15.00	District Council.	Placement as part of Advanced Certificate in Public Health. To gain knowledge of public health practice.	Health Promotion Specialist; Chief Environmental Health Officer.	Observed partnership meeting of an alliance of smoking and health. Met councillors and discussed changes.
15.00 to 17.00	Clinic (base).	Preparation for YMCA out-reach project.		Preparing sexual health material and lesson plans.
NURSE B				
8.00 to 14.00	Secondary school.	BCG immunisations and follow-up for absentees. Planning, implementing and evaluating the session.	Students and parents of absent students.	Planned session. Follow-up of students who had heaf test the previous week.
14.00 to 15.30	Office based.	Contact with health visitor about referral of vulnerable children transferring into school.	Health visitor.	Referral of five vulnerable children.
15.30 to 16.30	Health Centre.	Clinical supervision.	School nurse team leader.	Planned clinical supervision session.
NURSE C				
8.30 to 12.15	Secondary school.	BCG immunisation.	Year 9 and 10 pupils. Staff.	Planned.
13.15 to 14.30	Health Centre.	Letters about home visits. Phone calls regarding children with continence problems. Answering phone calls.	Parents of primary school pupils.	Needed to be done.

TIME	LOCATION	ACTIVITY	CONTACT WITH	COMMENTS
NURSE D				
09.00	School I.	BCG vaccinations.	Year 9 pupils.	Planned session following heaf test last week.
12.45	School II.	Issue emergency contraception.	Female pupil Year 9.	Following 9.15 phone call from pupil.
13.15	School II.	One-to-one.	Female pupil Year 8.	Planned appointment following a referral to social services and a home visit with mum last week.
13.45	School II.	One-to-one.	Female pupil Year 9 plus mother.	Follow-up planned meeting after A&E liaison. Health needs discussed.
14.15	School II.	Health Education – Relationships and introduction to contraception.	Class of 28 Year 8 pupils.	PHSE within SRE school policy, introducing sexual issues including condom demonstration.
15.15	In car.	Phone call from social services re a referral.	Social services duty team leader.	Discussion of expected outcomes of recent referral.
15.25	School III.	Drop-in clinic.	Any pupil.	For advice, information, support, emergency contraception, pregnancy testing.
16.30	Home visit.	One-to-one with child and discussion with parent re concerns.	Primary school pupil aged 8.	Discussion of child's possible depression and referral to CAMHS.
NURSE E				
A.M.	Clinic.	Clerical: Comcare, travel claim.		Usually team meeting on Monday morning.
.	Local refuge (women's).	Visiting family with 2 boys with behavioural difficulties.	Mother and grandparents.	

TIME	LOCATION	ACTIVITY	CONTACT WITH	COMMENTS
NURSE E (continued)				
A.M. (cont.)	School.	Delivered more BCG forms.	Nurses at the sanitorium.	More forms required before school breaks up for Easter.
P.M.	Clinic.	Met up with school health clerk in preparation for screening a child (height, weight, vision and hearing) who was absent when her cohort was seen.	Secretary at school to ask if child present.	Yes – child screened at primary school. Child previously known to social services.
	Clinic.	Telephone call.	Clinic nurse at CAMHS service.	School nurse and CAMHS are working jointly to support a family with previous social services input.
NURSE F				
8.30 to 11.15	Office based.	Dealing with post; organising audio clinic (member of staff responsible for this sick).		
		Arranged Care Planning meeting for diabetic child (primary age).	Parents to check on current position (telephone); specialist diabetes nurse/head teacher/parent.	Date/venue agreed over telephone. Drafted letter to send as confirmation.
11.15 to 12.00		Travelling.		
12.00 to 15.00	Health Centre.	Team Leader meeting.	Head of School Counselling Service. Other Team Leaders.	Overview of service development, referral routes/forms. Useful updating. Briefing on developments. Sharing information etc.
15.00 to 16.30	Health Centre.	Clinical Supervision.	Supervisor.	First session. Ground rules. Discussed sensitive issue. Service Level Agreement in Secondary School.
16.30 to 17.15		Travelling.		

TIME	LOCATION	ACTIVITY	CONTACT WITH	COMMENTS
NURSE G				
8.00 to 10.00	Base.	Answering telephone enquiries; dealing with paperwork.	Parents, schools, colleagues.	Queries regarding vaccination programmes, missed vaccinations. Planning Health Education sessions.
10.00 to 11.45	Key Skills Training Services.	Information visit re forthcoming school leaver boosters. Opportunistic health education re testicular self awareness and breast awareness.	Year 10 pupils. 16+ coordinator.	The pupils who attend this service are on roll in school but escorted, to a minimal extent, off-site. The schools pay a charge for their pupils to take up these places. 16+ clients have left school.
12.00 to 13.15	School.	Liaison with 16+ coordinator re focusing health education work. See 2 girls with eating problems. They requested to see 2 other pupils for different reasons.	Student receptionist. Attendance officer. 4 pupils.	Unplanned visit which was highly successful. The school was about to contact me to come and see a pupil.
13.15 onwards	Base.	Updating records, arranging vaccinations and session for key skills.	Parents. Clerical staff.	Not enough hours in the day.
NURSE H				
9.00	School.	Health assessments.	Year 1 pupils.	12 children seen in morning.
12.00	Health Centre.	Filing school notes; typing BCG forms; organising enuresis clinic; various telephone conversations with parents/teachers.		

TIME	LOCATION	ACTIVITY	CONTACT WITH	COMMENTS
NURSE I				
9.00	Health Centre.	Post, telephone calls, paperwork.		
12.00	Health Centre.	Team Leader meeting.	Other Team Leaders.	
NURSE J				
A.M.	Office based.	Liaison; message taking and response documentation.	Health visitors, school nurse, clerk.	This team has two bases. It is therefore important to preserve good links and communication between staff and bases.
P.M.	Health Centre.	Team Leaders meeting.	Team Leaders, coordinator, school counsellor.	Update, directives, commendation communication.

The diaries reported only on one day in the life of the school nursing service as experienced by ten nurses with differing roles and responsibilities. They do, however, demonstrate the wide range of activities undertaken by school nurses and the considerable amount of travel that they undertake. It was apparent that immunisation was still taking up much school nursing time, but that conducting drop-ins, consulting individual pupils and/or their parents, undertaking group work and teaching on 'growing up' and sexual health issues, providing support and advice for teachers and other professionals, preparing for and holding clinics, and administrative tasks, also figured strongly.

Northern study area 1

This location was the 59th most deprived local authority in the country with 12 wards among the 10 per cent of most deprived wards in the country. Unemployment was twice the national average, educational attainment levels were well below the national average, and teenage conception rates were high. A school nursing review carried out by the NHS Trust in 2000 identified the main areas of health need as the promotion of healthy lifestyles and healthy schools, child and adolescent mental health, chronic and complex health needs, and vulnerable children and adolescents.

The population of young people between 4 and 19 years in local authority schools was around 36,500. The location as a whole was divided geographically into three local areas, with a team of school nurses in each. Interviews were held with the Clinical Lead for School Nursing as well as nurses attached to the two case study schools.

A service in transition

The school nursing service in this location was also very much in a state of transition. A review of the service had been carried out in 2000 to look at provision and how it met both demands on the service and the policy agenda. Among its findings, the review had concluded that the service was to a large extent crisis driven. There was a very limited school nursing provision, and 88 per cent of nurses worked over and above their contracted hours. Mainstream school nurses had been overwhelmed by immunisation campaigns that had taken up 66 per cent of nursing time over the review period. They had had difficulty providing an accessible and responsive service because of a lack of time and large caseloads.

The increase in children with behavioural and mental health needs, and the need to provide practical and emotional support to vulnerable children and families, made the role more difficult, especially when most school nurses were unavailable during holidays. There was also an inequitable provision of service across the city. Overall, the review indicated that there was greater accessibility to, and satisfaction with, the service provided by special needs nurses than by the mainstream school nurses. There was also no clear career structure for the school nurses and links with services other than education were poor. The report noted that:

> 'School nursing was seen as an add on to other services such as health visiting and seen to be the poor relation.'

Nonetheless, surveys of parents, young people, and education staff (teachers and education welfare officers) indicated an appreciation of the service by those who had used it.

Among the recommendations of the review, which encouraged a public health role for the service, were a reduction in time spent on immunisation by creating a city-wide dedicated team of nurses to carry out this role, the further development of partnership work with education and other agencies, a focus on four priority areas identified by the review, a strengthening of multi-skilled teams led by school nurse practitioner specialists, increased work at the strategic level, and significant changes to working hours and working patterns.

Current directions within the service

Many new service developments were under way at the time of interview in response to these recommendations. One change was to the structure of the area-based nursing teams to prevent, as had happened in the past, situations where nobody could carry on a specific area of work if a nurse with particular skills left. The new strategy was, first, to encourage individual nurses to develop specialisms and, second, to set up teams with team leaders. These team leaders would then work closely together to help to ensure that good practice was shared between teams and across the city.

> 'So their role, if we get these team leaders, would be partly as practice teacher. They would teach people how to do this and how to go about it.'

Other structures designed to facilitate the transfer of good practice across the city included the establishment of a forum of school nurses that met about once a term. The purpose of this forum was to discuss innovations in nursing practice and to carry out informal mutual training:

> 'No matter what they told you in the classroom, when you're faced with it it's a different practice.'

As well as structures to facilitate the transfer of good practice across the city, the location was also examining and experimenting with new ways of working. Several new initiatives were under discussion. One was a funding bid to carry out an action research project to look at school nurse input within community contexts. The proposal was to employ one full-time and one half-time nursery nurse to work under a school health supervisor within a primary school, the family centre, and the local youth and play centre, to help parents understand the developmental needs of their children. The project would work with children in school, invite parents to the family centre to attend classes, and encourage children to go to the youth and play centre in their free time.

An extensive review of sex and relationships education was also being undertaken. Discussion within a multidisciplinary group that included youth and play workers, teachers, and those involved in family planning, health education and school health, was considering curriculum input for pupils from reception class all the way through to secondary school. New health clinics were being set up in a number of local schools, and encouraging young people to join summer schemes to prevent them getting into trouble during the long holidays was on the agenda.

Although nurses worked mainly within schools, and between school and home for primary-age pupils, there was a general move out into the community. Working with parents through community centres was a new development. This recognised that the public health role meant helping others to support themselves and their families rather than providing a comprehensive service. Working collaboratively was all part of this general strategy.

> 'No one group can deal with all the different problems in a vast population. And it is important to link in with the community policy … So we're listening and talking and I think that's what it's basically all about.'

Communication was important, if not always easy.

> 'I would say our biggest job is not talking to people in education in the schools, it's talking to the local education authority … We've got to move more closely to say "Will you please work with us and not just see education as the curriculum. There are other parts of the curriculum that we can add to where we have the skills."'

Overall, however, things were changing in many ways. In the past, school nurses had had a very bad image:

> 'People would say "Well, what do they do? They just work 9 to 5 and go to see kids and then they have the half term off". And, you know, Nitty Nora springs to mind and all those sorts of things! We did have a terrible image.'

Already school nurses were becoming better regarded within the health service as well as by the schools, pupils and parents they were in contact with. The recent change in title to school nurse advisors had helped to give them a better profile, partly because this stressed that nurses were not in school to take the role of first aiders and deal with children who had been sick or had fallen over.

'I think the message is getting across that we are there to
advise about health in its broadest sense.'

The Clinical Lead for School Nursing added that she had been heartened by
the recent *School nurse practice development resource pack* (Department of Health
2001) where, for once, 'we were not an add on'.

The mainstream school nurses

School nursing services were divided into two separate services in this northern
study area – the mainstream school nursing service and the specialist school
health nursing service. This meant that the mainstream school nurses did not
have any responsibility for pupils with physical disabilities, but might work
alongside the specialist school health nurses within schools. There was also a
learning disability team, not located within school health services, which was
multidisciplinary and comprised nurses, psychologists, a social worker, and
others. In addition, there was one child and adolescent mental health specialist
nurse in each of the three areas. These supported school health staff in
undertaking assessments and dealing with referrals. The mainstream school
nurses were the focus of the present study.

The school nurses in this study area were called school health advisors. There
were around 28 in post altogether around the city, and the total staffing
represented an equivalent of 18.45 posts including the support workers. In
addition to providing a service to the local authority schools these nurses did
have a limited health input within private schools to carry out all the BCG
immunisation and offer boosters to school-leavers. Although most nurses
worked only during school hours and term-time, there were some full-time
nurses in the location. Developments were currently under way to establish
more flexible hours of working to allow nurses to work during the holidays and
encourage the more vulnerable children to join play schemes or other activities.
The view was:

'So no, it shouldn't be 9 to 4 and every half term you're off.
You need to be there to be doing things.'

The nurse attached to one of the case study schools did work all year round.
She was about to change her role and transfer to a new school that would
replace two existing schools. She would be spending 60 per cent of her time in
the new school, i.e. all morning four days a week and all day once a week. She

had a G grade post and would have an F grade nurse to work with her. Their joint caseload would include four middle schools and another high school. The nurse was well known in her current school and expected to continue to have a high profile. She welcomed the extra hours she would spend in the new school and felt she would offer a good service. She explained how:

> 'A lot of the stuff we do is fire fighting. We respond to crisis. It is crisis intervention. What will be exciting about the new school is because you are there every day, because you have the time, you will be able to do more proactive stuff than reactive. I think a lot of stuff around health with young people … is the relationship stuff and just the drip messages all the time. You can't do that quickly. It has to be over a period of time to have any impact.'

The other case study nurse had been a school health advisor at a large school located on two sites about a mile apart for the previous four years. Although some visits had been brief, she had visited the school about four times per week during the previous month. She had a degree and an F grade post. Her caseload included five primary schools.

Asked about her profile, this school nurse was more concerned about her image among school staff than pupils. She said it was hard work making her presence felt and encouraging teachers to take up the services offered. She told how:

> 'It's a very nice school to work in. But I think when you're working, as all school nurses do, in somebody else's area, you've constantly got to be promoting yourself … I mean I turn up at meetings that I think I would have a good input to but I might not have been invited to, and they're always apologising, saying "Sorry, we didn't think". I think sometimes they've got to be like that really because teachers are like every other person – they've got an enormous amount of work to go through. They're constantly getting a new agenda.'

Formal service level agreements were not generally used in the study area, although there would be consultation between nurses and schools on services to be provided. Governors would be involved where necessary, such as if there was a decision to be made on whether to provide emergency contraception at a school.

Determining priorities

Despite a general philosophy that a limited service had to focus on the most vulnerable young people, however these might be defined, it was apparent that priorities and ways of working were currently very much under discussion. Evidence of value and effectiveness seemed to be very important in influencing future directions.

> 'So we've really clearly got to define what we're doing and why we're doing it. Things are done because historically they have always been done. Well, okay, fine, but who is benefiting from this? … And it is so incredibly difficult to prove very much.'

The value of innovations websites, and the recommendations of the National Institute of Clinical Effectiveness, were mentioned in this context. It was evident that being able to provide a needs-led service was crucial. Identifying and highlighting need was important not only in relation to the philosophy of the service, but also because this provided a case for extra resources. It also helped the service to further develop its public health role.

School profiling, which was beginning to be undertaken in the locality, was useful in this context, particularly as it took young people's views into account. As a first phase, a young person's health survey was being carried out with pupils in Year 9 at several schools across the city. This survey was likely to be extended to all schools in due course. Modelled on the Huddersfield survey (see page 75), the purpose of the exercise was to identify the health needs of individual schools, contribute to individual School Health Plans, and provide the basis for differing inputs by the school health team at a local level. Topics covered by the survey were general health; use and knowledge of the school health service; drugs, alcohol and smoking; food choices and weight control; feelings and emotions; sexual health; and environment and safety.

Priorities for the local school nursing service were, nonetheless, in practice dictated by many factors. The Clinical Lead for School Nursing summed up the service overall by saying

> 'It's about being reactive a lot of the time but also proactive and reactive all at once. And all that within the context of limited resources and competing priorities.'

School nursing in the case study schools

There were two case study schools in this area, and nurses at both reported that carrying out immunisation was important but time-consuming, and interfered with projects and other initiatives. One gave a detailed account of the complicated process involved. This began by finding convenient dates and a suitable room to carry out the programme, liaising with caretakers to make sure the hall would remain free, making a presentation to pupils to let them know what would happen, bringing in consent forms and distributing these to form teachers, taking responsibility for getting these forms back (which might mean another presentation at assembly), ordering vaccine, syringes, needles and so on, and booking a team of nurses for the dates in question. Equipment also had to be carted round in cars, and nurses had to get to school early on the appointed days to set up everything. There was then paperwork to be completed by school clerks, and pupils to be found on the day. Much clearing up remained, and there were usually follow-ups tasks such as discussions with concerned parents.

Immunisation programmes did, however, have spin-offs. They could be a good way to get to know pupils and they gave a chance to pick up on pupils' problems. The immunisation sessions could also be used as an opportunity to put out health information leaflets and posters.

In both case study schools only limited screening was carried out, generally for pupils identified as vulnerable as well as for some new entrants. Neither nurse had an input into the curriculum at the time of the interviews, but both had plans to do so and both were involved in educational projects in the locality. One hoped to be able, in the future and with assistance from other school nurses, to provide some input for each class in every year group. At the time she was helping to plan a health project where a team of nurses and youth workers, and probably a health promotion worker, would undertake a 'carousel morning of workshops' for sixth formers on sexual health and young adult well-being. Six workshops would address health issues such as sexually transmitted infections, pregnancy and terminations, well women and well men, breast and testicular examination, relationships and rights within these, and homophobic bullying.

The other nurse was considering future curriculum input but was daunted by the size of the school. With 12 classes in each year group, she would have to offer each session 12 times – and still provide only one session for one year group. She was currently working on a local project to develop a pilot sex and relationships education curriculum for pupils aged from 4 to 18 years. This would be rolled out locally and, if successful, throughout the city.

Providing a listening ear was an important part of the role of both nurses. At one school the nurse saw young people, including many pupils from the school, at a drop-in clinic located just outside the school premises. This facility operated after school once a week and was also staffed by a family planning doctor and a family planning nurse. The nurse also saw pupils one-to-one in school.

The second case study school was on a split site and drop-in sessions were held in each location once a week. There were two sessions at the larger site, one for the sixth form and one for younger pupils. The sixth form drop-in was not particularly well attended. The younger pupils, however, came in 'for anything' and talked about BCGs, their periods, diets, or anything else. There were some regular attenders, and about four groups of pupils usually turned up, which could be awkward if somebody else, who had not been before, was waiting for an appointment. The school was supportive of the drop-in and there were no problems if pupils were late for lessons as a result. The nurse worked alongside a family planning nurse at the other school site, and most of the Year 10 and 11 pupils who visited the drop-in wanted to discuss sexual health issues. The school did not have the facilities to prescribe the pill or provide emergency contraception, although the nurse had broached the issue with the school. She said:

> 'If we're supposed to be listening to what they're saying, this
> is what they're saying. [But] the school would have a
> problem, I think. They would worry about parents if we were
> actually seen to be providing that.'

The drop-ins collected information on contacts with young people together with the reasons for contacts. Over the period of one year, young people were most likely to attend the sessions to gain general information and advice, condoms, and sexual health advice. Others sought help with relationship and personal problems (Table 3.1).

Table 3.1 Pupils' reasons for visiting the drop-in at the case study school

	Years 7/8/9		Years 10/11		Years 12/13	
	April–July 2001	September–March 2001–2	April–July 2001	September–March 2001–2	April–July 2001	September–March 2001–2
Information and advice	30	97	8	25	13	13
Relationship and personal problems	8	21	4	16	8	1
Pregnancy test	0	0	3	6	1	3
Problems – home/school	0	1	0	2	0	0
Condoms	0	3	18	12	3	8
C-card	0	0	5	1	2	3
Emergency contraception	1	1	6	2	1	0
Sex health advice	0	9	7	16	4	3
Total	39	132	51	80	32	31

As an additional activity, one case study nurse planned to run a 'Health Shop' at lunchtimes when she moved to the new school. This would be set up in a specially fitted corner in the new 'super-duper' restaurant. It would give her a visibility in the school and provide an opportunity to hand out information on health issues. Confidential appointments would also be arranged for pupils who wanted them. The second case study nurse was helping to plan an AwayDay for sixth form pupils as a response to four recent pregnancies at the school. This was particularly interesting in that it was making a special effort to target boys.

Monitoring and assessment

There appeared to be several ways in which the school nursing service in this study area was being monitored and/or assessed. First, school nurses kept records of their own activities, although it was unclear how useful these were. Second, there had been some consultation with young people who had completed evaluation sheets and question sheets about services they thought were useful and those they would like. This had led to the resiting of one service to a location young people preferred. Third, there had been a project to look at sex and relationships education in primary schools. Open evenings had been held and parents were invited to look at different literature and say what they liked and did not like.

Northern study area 2

This location adjoined the northern study area 1 and also had pockets of deprivation and a range of local issues and problems. The area as a whole comprised four localities and public health nurses had produced profiles to determine the local priorities for service provision (see below). One area, for example, was looking at supporting teenage parents, working with Sure Start, multi-agency work with mother and toddler groups, multi-agency sex education work, helping parents talk to their children, and providing toothpaste for babies.

In this area interviews were held with the Practice/Professional Development Lead for School Nursing and two school nurses working at the case study schools.

The direction of change

Services in this location were, as in the other study areas, very much in a period of change. At the time of interview the locality was one of four Department of Health funded Whole System Demonstration Sites. As part of this health visitor and school nurse development programme, four health visitors and five school nurses took on the role of change activists to 'make things happen'. Adopting a multi-agency approach, the strategy was to involve as many key workers as possible in identifying health needs in each locality, developing an action plan, and allocating funding. The service was moving towards a greater public health role and towards more work within the wider community outside school.

As a demonstration site, the school nursing service had received considerable additional money as well as the change activists. This had had a positive impact:

> 'It is great for us because we have had lots of support.'

It was acknowledged, nonetheless, that multi-agency change was complex and depended on much more than just resources. There seemed to be several guiding principles underlying the new developments. These included the need for clear objectives and corporate commitment as well as leadership and effective management of the change process. There was also an awareness of the need to listen to front line staff, and to promote new skills and knowledge for a new agenda. Working in and involving the local community was also highlighted: members of the local community were invited to join in meetings to give their views on what they thought was important and how they would like public health services to work with them. Tying in with government policies was also on the agenda, as was empowering staff. The Practice/Professional Development Lead for School Nursing said:

> 'Who knows what the future holds. I just think it is an exciting time to be working in school health because we have got investment that we have never had before. And I think our role is being recognised as hugely important in public health. And it is about not letting them fall into the river, it's pulling them out and stopping them jumping in the first place. It's a very exciting time and it's a great place to work.'

The public health nurses were responsible for identifying local need in conjunction with other agencies across the community, and one of the tasks of the change activists was to encourage colleagues to work together more closely. Expectations from the whole systems pilot were for visible changes to services (including a greater family and child centred public health role, less inequality, empowerment of front line staff, and the involvement of users), shared learning, and demonstrated effective use of resources. It was very much a location-wide exercise:

> 'One umbrella is the big thing. We are all going to work together.'

Staff structure and patterns of working

As part of the process of development and change, all school health advisors had been renamed public health nurses and all had been given grade G posts. Other grades were, however, to be introduced to ensure good skill-mixing within teams as a whole. Many but not all nurses worked full time. In addition, one or two schools in the location had school nurses based in the school for a set number of hours each week (e.g. 10 hours) that the schools paid for. Apparently this had made the nurses much more visible and seemed to be working well.

A recent task on the agenda had been to make caseloads across localities as equitable as possible. Changes had been made and there appeared to be general satisfaction with the outcome. It was mentioned, however, that a weighting tool and guidelines to help determine how cases should be distributed between and within teams would be valued.

Nurses in the study schools

One of the case study school nurses had worked at her school for two years but had recently left. While at the school, she had visited at least once a week for a weekly drop-in or to collect post and see anybody she needed to. She spent less time at this school than others on her caseload, in part because she perceived the others to be more receptive. She did not think many pupils at that school would have known who she was. She had a grade G post and had received a range of training. There were a further two secondary and four primary schools on her caseload.

The other case study nurse had been at her school for less than a year. She spent more time at the case study school than others and pointed out how her role varied enormously between schools. Three or more visits had been made to the school in the previous month. Again, she thought that not many pupils at the school would know her. Her post was also at grade G level and she had similarly undertaken a range of training. There were an additional two high schools, two primary schools and one specialist unit on her caseload.

In general, this nurse felt that the school did not especially need her. It had not taken up the services she had offered and she wished there was better communication between her and the school about her role.

The profile of school nurses was still a big issue in the study area as a whole. Their title had been changed once to school health advisor and might change again to public health nurses. It seemed difficult to get away from the old image of a school nurse, particularly with the general public. Much better progress had, however, been made with professional colleagues and schools.

Determining priorities

The school nursing service was using the Huddersfield model to gain young people's views on services, and findings would be used to develop individual health plans for all schools. As in Huddersfield, the service was targeting a one-year group. An evaluation of the process as a whole, including its impact (e.g. on teenage pregnancies), was planned.

Priorities were also influenced by research and clinical experience, and the philosophy was to develop only strategies shown to be effective. Routine medicals had been discontinued as evidence suggested they were not the best approach, and the main focus had shifted to the most vulnerable young people. Child protection was acknowledged as a huge commitment in the locality characterised by areas of high deprivation. Teenage pregnancy, dental health, mental health and parenting were also identified in all localities as high priorities. There was concern to ensure that all age groups received an input from the available services. Overall, the emphasis was clearly on providing a needs-led service, even if this was no simple task:

> 'I think without the support of the public health specialists that we have had and the investment that we have had, it would have been extremely difficult. But the support and training we have had from them has made it a lot easier because it has focused us, trained us and given us the evidence for providing these services.'

Providing a service

The two case study school nurses in this area spent rather different amounts of time on immunisation. For one, the immunisation coordinator for the school health team, it was a large and important part of her work. Nonetheless, it took up more time than she thought necessary, and she planned to suggest that BCGs were carried out in the first year of secondary school rather than the last year of primary school to reduce the number of schools to be visited. The other nurse, by contrast, felt that she could play a greater role in enrolling pupils for the vaccination programme. There had been a very low take-up for the Diphtheria, Tetanus and Polio vaccination at her school, and she said she had not been given the opportunity to highlight its importance in assembly. She was anticipating an outcry from parents as they realised that their child had not been vaccinated although, in her words

> 'There is only so much you can do and you can't organise a school.'

No routine full-scale screening was carried out by school nurses in these case study schools. Both had had some limited input into the curriculum. One nurse had provided information on contraception and first aid, and also run a session on the role of the school nurse. She would have liked to spend more time on this activity, but wished schools would give more notice when they requested input. Lessons on contraception had been carried out with Year 9 pupils at the other school. The nurse had hoped to do a session on sexually transmitted infections, but there had not been time. She expected to carry out a role play exercise with pupils on visiting a sexual health young person's clinic in the near future.

A young people's clinic had recently been opened within one of the schools. This had previously been located in a temporary building opposite the school, and was run by the health authority with input from a family planning nurse and a family planning doctor. The school nursing service was not involved in this provision. The nurse did, however, hold a weekly session in a local family planning clinic attended by pupils from the school which helped her meet and keep in contact with these young people. In the past she had run a drop-in session at the school, but this had been discontinued. Since the sessions stopped, she had been meeting pupils either at the school or at her office. She would also see pupils at school about once a fortnight for child protection and other issues.

An irregular drop-in was held at the second school, but cancelled if other priorities intervened. The nurse said she was more likely to contact pupils informally than see them at drop-ins. She would like to spend more time providing a listening ear for pupils.

Among other activities, one of the nurses ran a weekly after-school girls' group, mainly for Years 7, 8 and 9, with a youth worker and two learning mentors. The group discussed health issues and held activity nights focusing on topics such as beauty therapy and aromatherapy. The nurse said

> 'It is really to get over to the young people that health
> doesn't have to be salad and going to the gym … It's a
> hugely successful group that I'm very proud of.'

One nurse also mentioned her involvement in a sexual health partnership coordinated by a local university, a drug education project alongside a voluntary organisation, and a local drug education team. She also pointed to the work she was carrying out with the teenage pregnancy coordinator.

Monitoring and record keeping

In line with an emphasis on research and clinical practice, there was recognition of the importance of monitoring and assessment. The current view was:

> 'We need some evidence to base our practice on because in
> the past we've never had this, and we think this might work.'

At the moment the service was looking at ways to keep meaningful statistics. This was hampered, however, by the lack of computer facilities. Despite the time spent on administrative tasks, few formal records were kept of school nursing activities. Details of child protection cases were kept, but these might be little more than a note of the date and name of pupils seen with further details only if necessary. Nurses did not recall any assessment or evaluation of the work carried out by school nurses in the school, but one thought this would be valuable:

> 'I've always thought that, perhaps at the end of term, we should be saying "This is what we've done this year". But we've never actually done that, so there's no real record of what you're doing and whether you've capitalised on what you've done during the year or bettered it, or whether it was worth it. But I think it's something we should be doing.'

She also reported that no feedback was given to schools or teachers unless asked for.

4.   Which way forward?

Pupils' views and experiences, and illustrations of the school nursing service, have been presented in earlier parts of this report. Here, they are brought together to highlight several key issues. School nursing has changed markedly in recent years but there remain challenges for its future direction if the needs of young people are to be best met.

A public health agenda

The evidence from this study suggests that the school nursing service is moving rapidly from a largely medical model to a much broader public health role. This means not only a different ideology and perspective, but also a shift in the day-to-day tasks a nurse might expect to undertake. The service in the two study areas had, generally speaking, embraced this new public health role with enthusiasm and there was an impression of innovation and change tempered only by the struggle to fit new initiatives alongside existing obligations. Nurses outlined key aspects of this new role:

> 'I think mainly at the moment the public health goal is about partnership work and, ultimately, whether … we are perceived to be the motivators and the visionaries.'

> 'Historically, practice used to be very universal. It was around universal screening at set ages … The way that the service has developed, especially locally, is that it has become far more proactive … We've moved from a reactive response to health promotion and parent empowerment.'

'It is far more about prevention, not just about prevention with the individual but around prevention with groups of young people. So it's targeting a school where there is a high number of children at risk as opposed to working with the individual.'

There was, nonetheless, a difficulty in maintaining the correct balance.

'I think there is a bit of a danger with school nursing that we go chasing every new initiative. Because we are a very small service we are almost fighting for our survival and management go round trying to tack us onto anything because in a sense it's almost our survival mechanism. Sometimes I feel it would be better to be more focused ... I think school nursing has perhaps tried to dissipate itself too much and that we should perhaps have a more realistic view of what we can do in the present with the resources we've got.'

There was also frustration, expressed by almost every nurse interviewed, at the disproportionate amount of time spent carrying out immunisations, dealing with messages, and undertaking administrative tasks.

'It is the proactive work, it's the moving the service forward, that I feel really suffers.'

The RCN School Nurses Forum (2002) evaluation of the Meningitis C immunisation programme highlighted how the campaign affected and undermined the work of the school nursing service in the UK, and this was universally corroborated by the nurses in the present study. A survey of RCN members had found that 97 per cent reported that the campaign had affected their normal workload, with 35 per cent stating that it had 'almost completely taken over their normal work'. The following comment is typical of what the nurses in this study said.

'I think most of the school nurses have found it frustrating in that you're trying to look innovatively to set up different projects and then immunisations come up, like the BCG ... and everything has to go on hold. I've certainly been to multidisciplinary meetings where you're trying to work together where that's been thrown back at me: "You haven't been able to come to this because you've got an immunisation session" or "We didn't include you because we know you're busy with immunisations".'

In summary, services were changing and taking on many of the requirements of a public health role. There were, however, obstacles in the way of moving forward and possible solutions, such as different arrangements for carrying out immunisation programmes, were under discussion. In the meanwhile services seemed characterised by both old and new models of working.

Determining need and determining priorities

The public health role carries with it the expectation that practice will be needs-led. So while it provides the potential to address a wide range of health issues facing children and young people, it does at the same time impose the necessity to establish what local priorities might be.

School health profiles are widely recognised as a valuable method of providing the local information required for determining a needs-led service (Bagnall and Dilloway 1996; Mosely 2002). At their most detailed, they combine data at school level with information on individual pupils and can pinpoint variation in health needs both between and within schools. They have the value of enabling school health services to be targeted more effectively and make the best use of limited resources. They can also, by providing essential baseline data, be useful in monitoring change. School profiles can also inform wider community profiles, such as teenage pregnancy strategies, health improvement programmes, and public health reports. They can be used to negotiate service level agreements between schools and school health services and contribute to effective collaboration between health and other agencies.

A well-publicised example of school health profiling is provided by the Huddersfield NHS School Nursing Service. This recently produced its second multi-agency school health profiles that can be viewed at district and PCT, individual school, or individual pupil level. Profiles include the main indicators that impact on the health of school-age children, such as drug use, sexual activity, accident and crime statistics, and mental health, and information is collected from partner agencies as well as young people themselves. Huddersfield has used profiling to help inform the local children's health improvement programme's priorities, targets within the local healthy schools programme, and school nurse health plans. It has enabled services to prioritise health needs and formulate public health programmes that are evidence-based, structured and evaluated (Mosely 2002).

Lightfoot and Bines (1996) reported that only a quarter of the school nursing services surveyed were regularly completing school health profiles, and this study too found that most schools and nurses did not carry out any kind of systematic profiling. The northern locations were, however, using the Huddersfield model referred to above. Even without formal profiling, however, school nurses generally felt that they had good knowledge of their local communities and were well aware of local priorities and needs.

It seemed that the study areas had priorities in theory and priorities in practice, and that these did not always match. All areas, teams and individual nurses had views on the most pressing local concerns but, in reality, were often unable to respond to these. Sometimes it was a question of time and resources, sometimes the cooperation of schools, sometimes the interests and expertise of local nurses, and sometimes the necessity to react to 'crisis' or meet an obligation such as immunisation. The general lack of conscious or well-developed practices of priority setting was an additional factor. Service level agreements in the southern study area were proving useful in helping to examine priorities and determine appropriate levels and types of contact with individual schools.

Meeting young people's needs

An important question for school nursing services is the extent to which they meet the needs of young people. Two issues arise. First, are young people's views being sought? And, second, if they are, what do they suggest?

It was encouraging to find from the present study that exercises had been carried out, or were planned, to gain feedback on services from young people. A nurse in the southern study area had helped to carry out a survey of young people some time ago to find out what they thought of existing services and what they would like, but said there had been no formal consultation since. Another nurse could not recollect any pupil consultation on school nursing at school. However she had received informal complaints from pupils saying they had asked for Saturday afternoon clinics and emergency contraception at school but nothing had happened. A third nurse hoped that the service level agreement with her school might include seeking pupils' views on the school nursing service, and the fourth was planning to give pupils questionnaires on their needs, their perceptions of her role, and how they thought she might help.

More systematically, a young person's health survey pilot study had been carried out in northern study area 1 with Year 9 pupils in five schools across the city. The two case study schools in this area reported additional surveys of parents and young people. One exercise had had a real impact. Young people had been unhappy about the location of a service, and it had been relocated as a direct result of their comments. The nurse mentioned other ways in which pupils had been included in activities at school.

> 'I think we do try to involve pupils and young people. I've just recently had a poster competition with cash prize money for designing posters for the drop-in … [And] before we started the drop-in we had a questionnaire with Year 12 pupils about what services they would like. And I do, whenever I speak to them, constantly ask for their input in things like that.'

She thought that while some pupils appreciated this, others were busy and did not really take much interest in health until they had a problem themselves.

Pupils were also being involved in service development in northern study area 2. This school nursing service, too, had started to use the Huddersfield model to gain young people's views on services and develop individual health plans for schools. An evaluation of the process as a whole, including its impact, was planned.

At one school the impact of school nursing input into the curriculum was being monitored through a pupil questionnaire before and after a lesson on contraception. This asked about prior and subsequent knowledge, what pupils did and did not like about the lesson, what they wanted from the session, and their usual sources of information on sexual health. Unfortunately pupils had said they wanted single sex classes – which could not be arranged. The nurse was planning to feed her findings back to the school to make other staff aware of pupils' needs and views.

The pupil survey reported earlier (see Part 2) looked at health needs and expectations of the school nursing service. The findings suggested some priorities for service development.

First, pupils indicated why they might consult school nurses. The main areas mentioned were minor illness and sexual health. This was interesting as school nurses did not, in general, see minor health matters as within their remit. This did not, of course, mean that they could not be consulted on such matters during drop-in sessions held at school.

Second, pupils reported on whether or not they had concerns or difficulties they wanted help with. About one in 12 pupils overall indicated that they did. Whether or not this was an accurate figure, it did suggest that some pupils had unmet needs. Pupils were also asked what these needs might be. Healthy eating and weight problems were mentioned most often, followed by asthma and dyslexia, family problems, general issues such as relationship problems, and bullying. Puberty, appearance, getting fit, suicide, self-harm, help with an injury, eating disorders, drugs, smoking, sexual health, exam stress, and bereavement or illness in the family, were also cited.

Some pupils completing questionnaires added comments:

> 'I think that youths should know more about confidential counselling and we should know more about our school nurse and more information about telephone helplines and about our different problems.'
> *(Male, Year 10)*

> 'I think young people want to know about health etc., but can't go to the nurse in case they get seen to care and get taken the mick.'
> *(Female, Year 9)*

> 'I think that health and worries are important to talk about. I have many problems but don't know where to go.'
> *(Male, Year 7)*

> 'I think that we need a website on the Internet where children can visit and chat to a professional (anonymously) and get help with their problems.'
> *(Male, Year 9)*

These young people did not know who to ask for help, or wanted to ring a telephone helpline or visit a website but needed assistance. A flexible school nurse role could help to meet all these needs, either directly or by providing information on other sources of support. Although many school nurses undoubtedly do address these matters, it is apparent that there are some pupils who continue to fall through the net.

Do boys and girls need different services?

There was clear evidence from the pupil survey that boys and girls sought different kinds of help and support for problems and concerns they might have. Marked gender differences were found, with girls tending to favour talking to somebody about their difficulties while boys preferred to deal with problems more anonymously. Thus boys were more likely than girls to turn to telephone helplines and the Internet, while girls were more likely to seek out support through personal contact. These patterns were consistent across reasons for wanting help or information, and true both for support they might seek and support they had sought in the past.

In line with this tendency, girls were much more likely to say they would consult, or had consulted, school nurses. They were also more likely to know how to contact the school nurse. Although this might be because they took more trouble to find out, it does still indicate that 'advertising campaigns' focused on boys could be worthwhile. Somewhat surprisingly boys more often than girls said they would go to see their family doctor if they had a worry or concern.

These gender differences in accessing services have been commonly reported and are no new finding. They do nonetheless reinforce the challenge for the school nursing service to find ways to provide appropriate services that boys will access. Nurses in the present study were very concerned about the difficulties they faced in encouraging boys to take up their services, and one said she had only ever seen two or three boys at school. Issues, such as drugs, could often be overlooked as a result. According to one nurse

> 'The much lesser contact with boys through the drop-in is likely to mean that many problems are missed. Girls seem to have a much clearer view of accessing the service, and the boys who have come to see me are usually quite needy individuals who will present me with a whole list of physical symptoms but you are very aware that there is some other issue behind there.'

An attempt to get boys more involved in a health AwayDay for sixth form pupils, by holding it at the local football ground, was mentioned by one nurse. This was the only example of a service directed specifically at boys that was encountered during this research. Other studies have provided further suggestions. Allen (2003), for example, indicated ways in which services might be made more attractive to boys: school nurses in her study reported that boys were more likely to attend drop-ins if these provided activities they liked, such as snooker. DeBell and Everett (1997) pointed to the almost exclusively female workforce within the school nursing service and suggested that the introduction of male nurses might also help to encourage boys to seek information and support.

A school-based service or a service for school-age young people?

Comments from pupils suggest that a service that is really going to meet their needs must be flexible and provide options. Should, then, school nursing provide a school-based service or a service for school-age young people?

Traditionally, school nurses saw children and young people at school. They would visit periodically, to administer injections and inoculations or perform the role of 'nit nurse', and would see those in attendance at the time. More recently the emphasis has shifted and the new public health role is interpreted more broadly. The Department of Health (2001) guidance discussed the need to tackle the causes of ill health right across the school-aged population, in part because there are groups of vulnerable children, such as travellers, refugee children, excluded children, and those who move frequently, who are not consistently at school. DeBell and Everett (1998) concluded that the school nursing service should in future be designated as for 'children of school age', with an extended range of sites where school nursing was delivered. This has been incorporated within a public health strategy in which these authors explicitly acknowledged the special responsibility school nurses have for vulnerable children and young people.

> There should be universal access to the School Nursing Service for every school-age child and young person who wishes to see a health professional. Nevertheless, service delivery should be geared to equity of access.

The evidence collected from the present research demonstrated that most services were currently provided at school even if this was less a matter of policy than a matter of necessity or convenience. Curriculum-based work and immunisation programmes clearly needed to be undertaken in these settings, and the provision of one-to-one advice and support was usually seen as best given at school. Being in school was beneficial in promoting the visibility of the school nurse and ensuring the maximum opportunity for her and young people to get to know each other.

Nonetheless, there were strong arguments for basing some services within the wider community. Young people might prefer to seek advice somewhere more anonymous and, perhaps, more comfortable. Although there was no information on their reasons, a number of pupils in the present study did say they would prefer to get support and information outside school. Home was mentioned most often, no doubt reflecting a preference for parental help and support. Apart from home, the most favoured locations were a doctor's surgery and school. A number of other contexts were also mentioned, such as drop-in centres, telephone helplines, youth clubs, and the Internet.

Surveys carried out by school nurses supported the view that some pupils preferred to receive services out of school and out of school hours. One exercise, for instance, revealed that pupils wanted a clinic on a Saturday or Sunday afternoon. Drop-ins at the school were mostly at lunchtimes, and pupils said they did not like it when appointments extended into lesson times. As the nurse pointed out, young people are going to value a service only if it is 'realistic' for them. This was increasingly acknowledged. One nurse said:

> 'Roles are changing … We are providing a service for school-age children, not school children. So therefore that moves the focus some way from the school to delivering the service wherever school-age children might be. That then encapsulates excluded children, children in different units, non-attenders … [and covers] outreach, evenings and weekends.'

A flexible service was especially important in reaching certain groups of children and young people. One school nurse was involved in three small projects with pupils excluded from school. Another mentioned work in two holding centres for asylum-seekers, and in a women's refuge where primary school-age children lived. The problem of reaching traveller children was also mentioned.

Apart from isolated instances, nurses were not regularly seeing school-age children in out-of-school contexts. They were spending more time in the community, perhaps working with parents, or maybe seeing children for straightforward health issues (bedwetting, hearing problems) at clinics, but this was mainly for work with younger children. A more widespread service for school-age pupils within the community would present a significant challenge for advertising their services. This study has shown that most young people have little idea of provision even within their own schools. Finding out about activities in other settings is likely to be even harder.

In summary, it seemed that available resources meant, in the short term at least, that most school nursing services would continue to be provided at school or through home visiting. In a few instances, nurses employed around the year could also offer other types of provision during holidays. Other possibilities for the longer term fell within the wider public health remit and were under discussion within nursing teams.

Working in partnership with other agencies

Partnership working is central to the concept of a public health role. A broad range of tasks and activities can be carried out only if good cooperation exists between services and if there is a clear understanding of the differing roles of each type of provision. This means liaison with a range of professionals providing services for school-age children and teenagers, links with local health initiatives and, most importantly, good relationships with schools within the areas in which school nurses work. As outlined by the Department of Health (1999b):

> We want them [school nurses] to draw on their nursing knowledge and pastoral care experience to support policies such as the healthy schools initiative. We want them to help young people make healthy lifestyle choices, to reduce risk-taking behaviour and to focus on issues such as teenage parenthood. They need to work in teams in partnership with teachers, health visitors and others to provide integrated programmes of support and health promotion.

However, as has been pointed out by Kiddy and Thurtle (2002):

> There is no national mandate for practice, and therefore uptake of the principles underlying some of the [government] papers has been greater in some areas than in others.

DeBell and Everett (1998) highlighted how the nature of school nurses' involvement within the healthy schools programme was vague. Wainwright, Thomas and Jones (2000) stated that there was little evidence in the Teenage Pregnancy Strategy to support school nurses or evidence of which interventions might be effective. They also argued that the same could be said for other targets for young people's health behaviour such as smoking, diet and exercise. Lightfoot and Bines (1996) found more generally that the role of school nursing was very unclear and that there was a lack of consensus about its appropriate scope.

Some corroboration of these findings came from the present study. A nurse working at a school taking part in healthy schools told how she was not involved in the initiative:

> 'I think this is partly about the school not involving us, but I think there is also an issue about health promotion and the school nursing not working. You have actually got these two people employed by health and the [healthy schools] person is relating to a teacher who, I think, is involved in PHSE but whom I have never met or heard of. So we are very much working in isolation.'

It was clear from the present research that study areas and nurses valued the concept of partnership working and included this among their aims. The Action Plan for 2002–2005 within the southern study area, for instance, outlined how school nurses worked closely and collaboratively with other health professionals in both primary and secondary care. GPs and community paediatricians, CAMHS and the school counselling service, education (family liaison officers, teachers, SENCOs), the Health Promotion Unit (especially the NHSS team and healthy schools nurses), sexual health services, the PSA coordinator, Sure Start, the Children's Fund, and parents, children and young people, were among those listed. Partnership work was also central to the new directions being taken by school nursing services in the northern study areas.

It was more difficult to determine the range and extent of contacts that occurred in practice and, without good knowledge of both local needs and the range of local services, no assessment could be made of the effectiveness of local services as a whole. There was an impression, nonetheless, of considerable variability in the inter-agency contacts of individual nurses and nursing teams. Some good examples of partnership working emerged, but these were not universal. The public health nurses in northern study area 2 were producing extensive local profiles and were also developing a database of deprivation and social exclusion covering health, income, employment, education, housing, transport and leisure at a borough, ward, and enumeration district level.

Working collaboratively with other agencies was key. Another nurse mentioned involvement in projects with the local university, a voluntary organisation, a local drug education team, and the local teenage pregnancy coordinator.

Partnership working can be easier in theory than practice, and the School Nurse Clinical Coordinator in the southern study area said:

> 'I think there should be much more multi-agency training, for example with social services, education. If you start to train people together at that level, they'll come with the same agenda, and know what each other's roles are. And they will respect and value each other, I think. But that's going to be very long term. As far as core training for school nurses is concerned, I think that some of our degree courses need to be modernised, I really do. They are not practice based, they're still very much on a medical model, the generic school nurse. That's not the way life is … And obviously training for specialisms has to be very much improved. Personally I think some of the training is becoming too academic – and that is stopping some nurses going for that training.'

Working with schools

Schools are perhaps the most significant partners for school nurses and it was apparent from the present study that such partnerships sometimes worked and sometimes did not.

A number of schools were extremely enthusiastic about the role of school nurses. A Deputy Head Teacher who valued the school nursing role said:

> 'Well we have gone through a period where we have had very little access to a school nurse. Now we've got a lot more access and it is a lot better now … We would like to use her resources in the curriculum so it's not just a service coming in and dealing with one or two youngsters, it's a service that stretches right across the school. We can then approach her for the knowledge that she's got and use that in a variety of ways.'

When partnerships worked well, nurses felt motivated and able to take the initiative in providing the kinds of services they thought were needed within the constraints of their own time and resources. When they did not work well, they felt considerable frustration and dissatisfaction.

> 'I don't think they [the teaching staff] fully understand my
> role but they haven't got the time to sit down and listen to
> what the role is. They are asking me for the wrong things
> like headlice situations. They are still asking me whether a
> child who has just fallen down has got a head injury. Well,
> where is your first aider? I am not the first aider!'

Ultimately, patterns of school nursing practice reflected the level of priority attached to health by different schools. According to the Children's Service Manager in the southern study area:

> 'It is tough in some schools … You can identify the issues
> but if the school doesn't want you to work with them, or they
> don't want to recognise the issue, then it is very difficult …
> That influences what we do in a way as well.'

Clear lessons emerged for what helped good relationships within a school. First, it seemed important that there was a proper and shared understanding on the services that could realistically be provided. Service level (or similar) agreements seemed particularly valuable in this context. Schools are formally required only to facilitate routine child-health surveillance and immunisation programmes, and agreement on the services to be offered was very useful, particularly in the area of sexual health. The Education Act 1993 gave school governors the power to decide whether or not to offer sexual health education, and decisions in this area could be sensitive and controversial. One nurse said of service level agreements

> 'I think it is part of putting our footing in a school on a
> more professional basis … I would also see the SLA as very
> much a way of trying to raise the profile of our service and
> to actually start a proper dialogue. I have also asked for a
> specific member of staff within the school that I could relate
> to, which again I hope will help.'

Another described how the agreement at her school covered all the input from the school nursing service, including the issue of emergency contraception, and was incorporated within school policy. Parents were made aware of it and the implications for how the school 'worked'. The nurse felt it was important that everybody was aware of what she was doing and not doing. She added:

> 'I'm sold now on packages of care. I suppose I feel that the service level agreement with the secondary school is almost a package of care. We're saying to them "In this school you can expect this from us and this is what we expect from you." And actually it works really well and that's what I'd like us to aspire to with the other secondary schools. It makes life so much easier if the governors know and if the parents know.'

A willingness on both sides to communicate exactly what each expected was, however, not always present. According to one nurse:

> 'When I started at this school I gave out details of what I anticipated my involvement would be to every year head and the key people in the pastoral head system ... I sent out documentation and things about what I would like to do .... Nobody really responded to that and then I got to the point where I sent letters in envelopes with stamps on and even asked to go to staff meetings. I got no feedback whatsoever from anybody.'

Practical considerations, too, affected the effectiveness with which the school nurse felt she could provide a service. A common lament was the lack of a suitable private room for a drop-in or one-to-one session with a pupil. Another was that pupils had to queue up to see her opposite the Head's room or in another prominent position. Such factors, even if beyond the control of teachers, were likely to affect take-up of her services.

> 'Accommodation makes a big difference and schools are very poorly accommodated. Every inch of space is taken and it's really quite difficult sometimes to actually establish a reasonable place to carry out services – even to carry out immunisations, never mind drop-ins.'

Last, but certainly not least, was the time nurses were allocated for contacts with young people in school. Very often, in the view of nurses, this was insufficient. It might mean inadequate time to provide an input into the curriculum, to hold drop-in sessions, or to talk to pupils and staff in other settings. On the whole individual nurses and individual schools negotiated the provision to be made by the school nursing service, and this might or might not be successful. Greater intervention from education departments at strategic level to facilitate effective communication might be valuable and could be one recommendation for the way forward.

The question of resources

Kiddy and Thurtle (2002) have argued that despite raising the profile of school nursing and linking it closely with the public health agenda

> There are few pointers as to how we are expected to achieve it within current resources … and most school nurses across the UK are concerned that the help they need to re-develop their role will not be available to them.

Certainly, the shortage of resources faced by the school nursing service was a recurring theme throughout this research. Two of the key issues were the size of the workforce and the restricted hours that many school nurses worked. The School Nurse Clinical Coordinator in the southern study area reported

> 'The problem for school nursing is that there has been no new investment in the service … Over the last ten years, the only new investment has been through healthy schools which is discrete separate funding. So every development we have made has been within existing resources. And of course taking on these big new roles, and developing roles within existing resources, [is difficult]. I did put in a bid this year for three public health nurses, but we were overspent and the financial position was not good and they said no.'

She pointed to the limitations of short-term funding which did not provide a proper opportunity to develop new skills and new initiatives. Money could sometimes be found for specific projects but this was often ring-fenced. A very practical implication of limited resources in the northern study area had been the lack of computers. In one office nurses had to produce materials or seek information on the Internet at home. This office did not appear to have even a fax machine.

Funding levels had direct implications for staffing levels. Current national rates of school nurses are not available, but there are fewer than 3,000 in the UK as a whole of which many work only part-time and most are employed only during term-times. This is a small number in relation to 8 million school-age children in England alone. The Court Report (Secretary of State for Social Services 1976) recommended that there should be one school nurse per 2,500 pupils, but as Bagnall and Dilloway (1996) demonstrated, this level was met in only half of all NHS Trusts (52 of 101) at the time of their study.

The shortage of school nurses for the populations they served was frequently highlighted in the study areas. The Children's Service Manager in the southern study area told how:

> 'We did an exercise. In the Strategy for Public Health there is a recommendation for minimum requirements and the minimum number of school nurses to population. I think it's something like a team of six school nurses for a population of 6,000. If we use that figure we need £250,000 to bring our service up to that level.'

One of the northern study areas had undertaken a review of school nursing services in Spring 2000 and concluded that the 'service is struggling to meet the demands – it is crisis driven'. Eighty-two per cent of school nurses worked over contracted hours, with 31 per cent working in excess of 11 to 19 hours extra per week, and whole teams working 3 to 37 hours between them in extra hours. Sixty-six per cent of staff time during the period of the review was taken up by the meningitis campaign. This review also calculated that school nurses were responsible for six to 16 schools and between 2,100 and 6,000 pupils.

Not only the number of nurses, but also the hours they worked, seemed important. Although things were changing, many nurses in the study areas were employed on term-time only contracts. This matched the national picture (CPHVA/MSF 2001). Most school nurses and their managers felt strongly that the service should operate for twelve months of the year. Some comments were:

> 'If I had a magic wand I would offer every school nurse we employ the opportunity to work all year round ... The number one priority is that we have year round cover, not only for the needs of the young people, children and

transition stage, but also for the profile of the service. We just disappear, so we need to maintain that cover for our credibility as well.'

'If the service was year round we would be more aware of the locality and community issues because we would have more time to look into that. We would be able to develop more links with other people, agencies and partners.'

'If kids knew that the drop-in sessions were maintained through the summer, they would be able to access those. I think that would be very important because there are some youngsters [who] need those services … It would be nice if youngsters could know that they could come to school and say "I need to see the school nurse". They don't just have health needs when school is open.'

'A lot of preparation could be done in the school holidays. Some teachers work during the school holidays, you know, they're in doing preparation work. There are Inset days too. You could be in school working with teachers.'

These findings have real implications for the size of the school nursing workforce. Nonetheless, optimal staffing levels cannot realistically be specified without taking account of the future role of school nurses, the services to be provided, the input from other agencies and professionals, and the degree of inter-agency partnership working. Practical and intellectual discussion of the interrelationship between all these factors would seem to be a high priority to inform the debate on the way forward for the service.

The profile of the school nurse

An enormous amount of enthusiasm, resourcefulness and optimism was encountered among the school nurses and their managers throughout the present research. The impression was that most school nurses enjoyed their job and put considerable energy and personal resources into carrying out their role as effectively and comprehensively as they could. This enthusiasm was, however, to some extent countered by factors relating to their profile and status within the community. Two issues that arose in this context were the clarity of the professional role and their job title.

The clarity of the school nurse role was a key issue. McConville (2002) stated that

> Today the government sees school nurses in a role that ranges from immunisation campaigns to citizenship training in schools, from personal health and social education to assessing the needs of communities, from promoting positive parenting to working in multi-disciplinary partnerships.

In many senses, this breadth of role is likely to contribute to the confusion that remains amongst many professionals in both health and education fields, as well as among parents and young people, about the services the school nurse provides and the skills and experience that she has (Lightfoot and Bines 1996; DeBell and Everett 1998). Findings from the present research reflected these concerns. The school nurses reported how they felt that the public at large had little idea of who they were and what they did. They were appreciated by those they worked with, but their small numbers meant they were not much noticed by anybody else. The point was also made that the wide range of professionals who now work in schools had made their role even less clear. There was not always a clear demarcation of tasks and there could be considerable overlap between the functions of different workers.

Evidence from the pupil survey confirmed the 'invisibility' of many school nurses. Although three-quarters of pupils said they knew who the school nurse was in the case study school with its own full-time school nurse, the story was quite different in the rest. In the five schools without an extra nurse, only one in six pupils said they knew who the school nurse was. Moreover, just over one in three knew how to contact her, and most did not seem to know when she would be in school. Over half the pupils said they had not received any information about her role and the service she provided. Two added:

> 'The school nurse should be promoted more around the school as I never knew we had one.'
> *(Female, Year 7)*

> 'I can only turn to some teachers, maybe just one. Some teachers don't take it seriously and some are not very good listeners. We should have a school nurse and school doctor here everyday.'
> *(Female, Year 10)*

The nurses themselves referred to the rather haphazard publicity they often received. The importance of being known was commonly stressed and it was clear that the school nursing service could have been better advertised almost everywhere. This applied to being known by other staff in school, by pupils and other young people, and by the community more generally.

More positively, things seemed to be improving. The public profile and perception of school nurses in the study areas had become much better in the last few years, partly because many school nurses were now graduates. The service as a whole was seen as far more professional and had lost its 'Nitty Norah' image. Working in the community more had also helped. Nonetheless it was an uphill task and involved school nurses in a considerable amount of self-promotion.

> 'When you actually talk about the other things that school nurses do, people sit back. Even professional colleagues sit back and say "I didn't know you did any of that". So I think we need to sell our service, we need to keep on selling our service, we need to highlight our service. And if people don't know about the service, it's really our fault.'

There has been much recent debate about the most appropriate title for members of the school nursing service, and this was ongoing within the study areas. Not all nurses were now technically called school nurses and, in some cases, a first change in title was already being superseded by a second. Decisions about the most appropriate title seemed to focus on the role of the professional worker (was she a nurse or was she really an advisor?) and the context in which she worked (was it important or misleading to include 'school' in her title?). There was also discussion on whether a nurse's specialism should be included in her title. In the southern study area the title School Health Advisor (as used in the northern study area) had originally been favoured, but this had since been changed to Public Health Nurse followed by any specialism in a bracket. The school nurses wanted to retain 'nurse' in their title but felt that 'school' should be dropped as much more work was being carried out within the community. This new title would, in addition to school nurses, cover district nurses and community children's nurses.

Monitoring and evaluation

A considerable amount of school nursing time was spent on administrative tasks, much of which involved keeping records of contacts with pupils, writing up notes on child protection cases, recording immunisations, writing referral letters, and maintaining pupil records. There was a clear recognition of the need for evidence-based services, and an appreciation that gaining additional resources was made easier if the nature and effectiveness of existing services could be demonstrated. How to keep meaningful statistics was an issue firmly on the agenda in the study areas.

The present research did not come across many examples of service evaluation in a more formal sense within the study areas. This seemed less because possibilities had not been considered than because there were many difficulties involved. Although immunisation was easy to audit and evaluate – uptake could be recorded and compared with the target – the same was not true for most other aspects of service provision. It was hard to know what impact a particular service had had and indicators in themselves did not necessarily help. The Children's Services Manager in the southern study area explained:

> 'I think the area that needs a lot of work on is around public health work and health promotion work. What is an outcome? Is it whether you have a process outcome or whether you have a long-term outcome? You've got an indicator for the reduction in teenage pregnancies. But you have no idea if your intervention has contributed to that or not … Maybe you've reduced it by 10 per cent and somebody else has increased it by 20 per cent.'

Curriculum input was similarly difficult to evaluate in terms of longer-term indicators. As one nurse pointed out, the best that can be done is to look in some way at attitudes or behaviour at the time, as you cannot wait years to see if there has been any impact on the teenage pregnancy rate or parenting. Another nurse talked about the babysitting course she ran and questionned how she could tell how many teenagers might consequently change their behaviour or choices.

How to monitor and evaluate provision in a meaningful and effective way was at once a priority and a challenge for the areas in the present research study.

In conclusion

The school nursing service is changing rapidly. Nursing teams and school nurses in the study areas were shedding the old medical model and taking on tasks enabling them to fulfil a much greater public health role. There was much enthusiasm and innovation and very real changes in provision were being effected.

The service nonetheless faced many challenges. It was, in the view of many, severely under-resourced, and it was struggling to combine the new role with the old. The statutory need to carry out immunisation programmes in particular was a task that severely interfered with much of the other work the nurses were hoping to undertake. The visibility of the school nurses, and general understanding of their role and the services they could provide, was also a matter of some concern. Most pupils at school did not know who their school nurse was, how they could contact her, or what she offered. Few young people suggested that she would be a first choice as a source of information and support.

There are challenges for the future of the service at many levels. At strategic level, there is a need for more resources to be made available wherever possible, as well as greater organisation of partnership working to encourage better and more appropriate use of a clearly overstretched service. School nurses operate more successfully at some schools than others. Less receptive schools should also receive greater encouragement to take up the services on offer. At school nursing level there needs, in turn, to be much greater cooperation and collaboration between agencies to ensure that joined-up working occurs between professionals. The continued development of a structured approach to the service provided that incorporates the identification of needs and priorities, systems of resource allocation, and increased levels of monitoring and evaluation, is also crucial. Alternative ways of dealing with immunisation programmes would be welcomed, and mental health issues facing pupils might then be accorded a higher priority. It was encouraging that services were beginning to listen more to what young people said they wanted and needed, and that these views were being used to inform service development.

The school nursing service also needs to be advertised much more effectively than at present so that schools and pupils realise what is on offer. Young people who have contacted and consulted school nurses are generally appreciative of the service they have received and, as witnessed by the case study school with its own full-time school nurse, will use such a service if it is well known and easily accessible. In other words, the low use of school nursing services is likely to reflect a lack of knowledge about what is on offer rather than simply an unwillingness to approach a school nurse.

It is important that the service moves on in all these ways as an outcome of debate, discussion and evidence, and with an appreciation of what is needed as well as an understanding of what is effective and realistic. A holistic view, which places the school nursing service within the wider context of alternative provision, partnerships and innovation, and which is underpinned as much by intellectual argument and demonstration as by precedent, preference and intuition, is the only way forward.

Finally, the school nursing service will be most effective if it is flexible. The move towards a public health role, the introduction of skill-mixing, the tentative moves out from the school into the community, the establishment of new initiatives to meet specific pockets of need, and a willingness to innovate, are all promising signs. Identifying need on an individual as well as a locality and school basis is also essential, as is the development and structure of services with both boys and girls in mind. The challenges are endless.

References

Allen, B (2003) *A qualitative study to explore school nurses' experience of running lunchtime drop-in in secondary schools*. Dissertation submitted to the Peninsula Medical School for the degree of Master of Science in Health Care

Bagnall, P (1997) The future contribution of school nurses to the health of school age children, *Health Education*, 4, 127-131

Bagnall, P and Dilloway, M (1996) *In search of a blueprint: a survey of school health services*. The Queen's Nursing Institute

Bagnall, P and Dilloway, M (1997) *In a different light: school nurses and their role in meeting the needs of school age children.* The Queens Nursing Institute

Balding, J (2001) *Young people in 2000*. Schools' Health Education Unit, Exeter

Balding, J (2002) *Young people in 2001*. Schools' Health Education Unit, Exeter

British Heart Foundation (2000) *Couch kids: the growing epidemic. Looking at physical activity in children in the UK*. British Heart Foundation

Burns, F (1999) Sexual and reproductive health of boys and men, *British Medical Journal,* 319, 1315-1316

Churchill, R et al (1997) *Factors influencing the use of general practice-based health services by teenagers*. Division of General Practice, University of Nottingham

Churchill, R, Allen, J, Denman, S, Williams, D, Fielding, K and van Fragstein, M (2000) Do the attitudes and beliefs of young teenagers towards general practice influence actual consultation behaviour? *British Journal of General Practice,* 50, 953-957

Clarke, M, Coombs, C and Walton, L (2003) School based early identification and intervention service for adolescents: a psychology and school nurse partnership model, *Child and Adolescent Mental Health*, 8, 1, 34-39

Coleman, J and Schofield, J (2001*) Key data on adolescence 2001*. Trust for the Study of Adolescence

Coleman, J and Schofield, J (2003) *Key data on adolescence 2003*. Trust for the Study of Adolescence

Cotton L, Brazier, J, Hall, DMB, Marsh, P, Polnay, L and Williams TS (2000) School nursing: costs and potential benefits, *Journal of Advanced Nursing*, 31, 5, 1063-1071

CPHVA/MSF (2001) *Making the grade. Grading guidance and the school nurses salary survey 2001*

Dawson, N (2002) *A short-term evaluation of TIC TAC (Teenage Information Centre/Teenage Advice Centre)*. Unpublished report

Day, P (2000) School nurses and contraception, *Nursing Times*, 96, 31, 39-40

DeBell, D and Everett, G (1998) The changing role of school nursing with health education and health promotion, *Health Education*, 3, May, 107-115

DeBell, D and Jackson, P (2000) *School nursing within the public health agenda: a strategy for practice*. Community Practitioners' and Health Visitors' Association, The Queens Nursing Institute and the Royal College of Nursing

Department for Education and Employment (1997) *Excellence in schools*. The Stationery Office

Department for Education and Employment (2000) *Connexions: the best start in life for every young person*. The Stationery Office

Department for Education and Skills (2001a) *Access to education for children and young people with medical needs*. Stationery Office

Department for Education and Skills (2001b) *Promoting children's mental health within early years and school settings*. Department for Education and Skills/ Excellence in Schools

Department of Health (1992) *The health of the nation: a strategy for health in England*. HMSO

Department of Health (1994) *Negotiating school health services*. HMSO

Department of Health (1996) *The Patient's Charter: services for children and young people*. HMSO

Department of Health (1999a) *Making a difference: strengthening the nursing, midwifery and health visiting contribution to health and healthcare*. HMSO

Department of Health (1999b) *Saving lives: our healthier nation*. HMSO

Department of Health (2000a) *National diet and nutrition survey: young people aged 4 to 18 years. Volume 1: Report of the diet and nutrition survey*. The Stationery Office

Department of Health (2000b) *Tackling teenage pregnancy: action for health authorities and local authorities*. Teenage Pregnancy Unit

Department of Health (2001) *School nurse practice development resource pack*. The Health Visitor and School Nurse Development Programme

Department of Health (2002) *Statistics on young people and drug misuse England 2000 and 2001*. Department of Health

Diekstra, RFW, Kienhorst, CWM and de Wilde, EJ 'Suicide and suicidal behaviour among adolescents' *in* Rutter, M and Smith, DJ *eds.* (1995) *Psychosocial disorders in young people. Time trends and their causes*. Wiley

Eliott, E, Watson, A and Tanner, S (1996) *Time to put the children first: children's and young people's views of health care in Salford and Trafford*. Public Health Research and Resource Centre, Report 7. University of Salford

Elliott, M *ed.* (2002) *Bullying. A practical guide to coping for schools. 3rd edition*. Pearson Education and Kidscape

Erens, B, Primastesta, P and Prior, G (2001) *Health survey for England: the health of minority ethnic groups 1999*. The Stationery Office

Farrell, C (1978) *My mother said....* Routledge

Gleeson, C, Robinson, M and Neal, R (2002) A review of teenagers' perceived needs and access to primary health care: implications for health services, *Primary Health Care Research and Development,* 3, 193-203

Gunnell, J (2000) Babysitters' club after school: a health promotion initiative, *Community Practitioner,* 73, 12, 873-874

Hall, DMB and Elliman, D *eds.* (2003) *Health for all children*. Fourth edition. Oxford University Press

Harris, B (1995) *The health of the school child: a history of the school medical service in England and Wales.* Open University Press

Harrison, H 'A child's view – how ChildLine UK helps' *in* Elliott, M *ed.* (2002) *Bullying. A practical guide to coping for schools. 3rd edition.* Pearson Education and Kidscape

Haselden, L, Angle, H and Hickman, M (1999) *Young people and health: health behaviour in school-aged children*. Health Education Authority

Hawton, K, Fagg, J, Simkin, S, Bale, E and Bond, A (2000) Deliberate self-harm in adolescents in Oxford 1985-1995, *Journal of Adolescence,* 23, 47-55

Hawton, K, Rodham, K, Evans, E and Weatherall, R (2002) Deliberate self-harm in adolescents: self report survey in schools in England, *British Medical Journal,* 325, 1207-1211

Health Development Agency (2002) *National Healthy School Standard: school nursing*

Jackson, C (1990) Homeless at school. Too few days in the school week, *Health Visitor,* 63, 6, 187

Jackson, P and Plant, Z (1997) Mock sexual health clinics for school pupils, *Health Education,* 1, 16-18

Jacobson, LD, Wilkinson, C, and Owen, PA (1994) Is the potential of teenage consultations being missed? A study of consultation times in primary care, *Family Practice,* 11, 3, 296-299

Johnson, A, Wadsworth, J, Wellings, K, Field, J, with Bradshaw, S (1994) *Sexual attitudes and lifestyles.* Blackwells

Jones, R, Coleman, J and Dennison, C (2000) *Community health initiatives for young people: a working paper.* Trust for the Study of Adolescence

Jones, R, Finlay, F, Simpson, N and Kreitman, T (1997) How can adolescents' health needs and concerns best be met?, *British Journal of General Practice,* 47, 631-634

Kari, J, Donovan, C, Li, J, and Taylor, B (1997) Adolescents' attitudes to general practice in North London, *British Journal of General Practice,* 47, 109-111

Kiddy, M and Thurtle, V (2002) From chrysalis to butterfly – the school nurse role, *Community Practitioner,* 73, 8, 295-298

Kurtz, Z and Thornes, R (2000) *Health needs of school age children: the views of children, parents and teachers linked to local and national information.* Department of Health and Department for Education and Employment

Lightfoot, J and Bines, W (1996) *Keeping children healthy: the role of school nursing.* Social Policy Research Unit, University of York

Lightfoot, J and Bines, W (1997) Meeting the health needs of the school-age child, *Health Visitor Journal,* 70, 2, 58-61

Lightfoot, J and Bines, W (2000) Working to keep school children healthy: the complementary roles of school staff and school nurses, *Journal of Public Health Medicine,* 22, 1, 74-80

Lightfoot, J, Mukherjee, S and Sloper, P (2001) Supporting pupils with special health needs in mainstream schools: policy and practice, *Children & Society,* 15, 57-69

Lightfoot, J, Wright, S and Sloper, P (1999) Supporting pupils in mainstream school with an illness or disability: young people's views, *Child: Care, Health and Development,* 25, 4, 267-283

McConville, B (2002) What's in a name?, *Health Development Today,* 7, 16-18

Madge, N (1997) *Abuse and survival: a fact file.* The Prince's Trust – Action

Madge, N and Harvey, J (1999) Suicide among the young – the size of the problem, *Journal of Adolescence,* 22, 145-155

Meltzer, H, Harrington, R, Goodman, R and Jenkins, R (2001) *Children and adolescents who try to harm, hurt or kill themselves.* National Statistics

Mental Health Foundation (1999) *Bright futures: promoting children's and young people's mental health*. Mental Health Foundation

Ministerial Group on the Family (1998) *Supporting families: a consultation document.* The Stationery Office

Mosely, H (2002) Building windmills: changing a service to meet the needs of a changing society, *Community Practitioner,* 75, 8, 286-288

Mukherjee, S, Lightfoot, J and Sloper, P (2002) Communicating about pupils in mainstream school with special health needs: the NHS perspective, *Child: Care, Health & Development,* 28, 1, 21-27

NHS Centre for Reviews and Dissemination (1997) *Preventing and reducing the adverse affects of unintended teenage pregnancies.*

NHS Executive (1996) *Child health in the community: a guide to good practice.* Department of Health

Ofsted (1996) *Exclusions from secondary schools 1995/6*. Stationery Office

Oppong-Odiseng, A and Heycock, E (1997) Adolescent health services: through their eyes, *Archives of Disease in Childhood,* 77, 2, 115-119

Osbourne, N (2000) Children's voices: evaluation of a school drop-in health clinic, *Community Practitioner,* 73, 3, 516-518

RCN School Nurses Forum (2002) *Evaluation of the 1999-2000 UK meningitis C campaign*. Royal College of Nursing

Reilly, JJ and Dorosty, AR (1999) Epidemic of obesity in UK children, *The Lancet,* 354, 9193, 1874-1875

Schofield, M (1965) *The sexual behaviour of young people*. Longmans

Secretary of State for Social Services (1976) *Fit for the future: the report of the committee on child health services (Court Report)*. HMSO

Wainwright, P, Thomas, J and Jones, M (2000) Health promotion and the role of the school nurse: a systematic review, *Journal of Advanced Nursing,* 32, 5, 1083-1091

Wallace, W (1999) Sex and the school nurse, *Nursing Standard,* 13, 36, 16-17

Wellings, K, Nanchahal, K, Macdowall, W, McManus, S, Erens, B, Mercer, CH, Johnson, AM, Copas, AJ, Korovessis, C, Fenton, KA and Field, J (2001) Sexual behaviour in Britain: early heterosexual experience, *The Lancet,* 358, 1843-1850

While AE, and Barriball, LL (1993) School Nursing: history, present practice and possibilities reviewed, *Journal of Advanced Nursing*, 18, 1202-1211

Yamey, G (1999) Sexual and reproductive health: what about boys and men?, *British Medical Journal,* 319, 1315-1316